FOR A BLISSFUL BABY

Dearest Anu & Ramu
with love
& wishing you the
best in life

Kumud
aunty
April 2011

For a Blissful Baby

*Healthy and Happy Pregnancy
with Maharishi Vedic Medicine*[SM]

by
Kumuda Reddy, M.D.
Linda Egenes, M.A.
Margaret Mullins, MSN, FNP

Samhita Productions
Schenectady, New York

Illustrations in Chapter 5 courtesy of Julia Preminger
Illustrations in Chapter 14 courtesy of Adam Schickling

Published by Samhita Productions
1537 Union Street, Schenectady, New York 12309
1-888-603-9171

ISBN 1-929297-01-7

We gratefully acknowledge permission to use material from the following pub-
lished sources. The charts and text on pages 11, 15, 18, 28, 29, 30, 37, 58, 99,
109, 113, 135, 144, 196, 218 and 219 are adapted from *Scientific Research on the
Maharishi Transcendental Meditation and TM-Sidhi Programs: A Brief Summary of
500 Studies* (Fairfield, IA: Maharishi University of Management Press), ©1996 by
Maharishi University of Management, from *Scientific Research on the Maharishi
Technology of the Unified field: The Transcendental Meditation and TM-Sidhi Program*
(Fairfield, IA: Maharishi International University Press), © 1988 by Maharishi
International University and from *Scientific Research on the Maharishi Transcenden-
tal Meditation and TM-Sidhi Program*, Vol. 3 and 4 edited by R. Chalmers, G.
Clements, H. Schenkluhn, and M. Weinless (Netherlands: MVU Press, 1990 and
1991), and Vol. 5 edited by R.K. Wallace, D.W. Orme-Johnson, and M.C.
Dillbeck (Fairfield, Iowa: MIU Press, 1991). The charts and texts on pages 58,
146, and 217 are adapted from *Summary of Research Findings* (Colorado Springs,
CO: Maharishi Ayur-Veda Products International, Inc.), 1996.

Printed in the United States of America.

With deepest gratitude to
His Holiness Maharishi Mahesh Yogi

Contents

Acknowledgments

We would like to thank Dr. Keith Wallace, Dr. Tony Nader, Dr. Nancy Lonsdorf, and Vaidya Hemant Gupta for their guidance and care in reviewing the manuscript; Susan Shatkin and Dick Kaynor for editing; Shepley Hansen for cover design; Julia Preminger and Adam Schickling for artwork; Craig Ridgley for typesetting; and Clara Berno and the other pioneers who helped make this knowledge available to thousands of mothers and their children.

A Note from the Authors:

The information included in this book is not in any way intended as a substitute for standard obstetrics or pediatrics. It is important that every woman follow the advice of her obstetrician during pregnancy, childbirth, and postpartum. Maharishi Vedic Medicine offers valuable complementary recommendations to supplement the advice of the primary care obstetrician.

Foreword

by Nancy Lonsdorf, M.D.
Medical Director
Maharishi Vedic Medical Center, Bethesda, MD

The deepest desire of all parents is for their children to be happy. This book will help fulfill that desire. It is about creating a more blissful baby and child through the time-tested knowledge of Maharishi Vedic Medicine. This ancient tradition of health care teaches that a child's physical, mental, and emotional life begins to be structured from the moment of conception—indeed, from even before conception—as a direct result of the health and happiness of the parents.

According to Maharishi Vedic Medicine, the key to creating a more blissful baby is first to create a more blissful parent, particularly a more blissful mom—a mother who feels nourished herself, even as she prepares to nourish her child. *For a Blissful Baby* could just as easily be called *For a Blissful Mother*, because it's essentially about nurturing the nurturer. For a balanced, healthy, and happy baby, the mother herself must radiate these qualities.

Unfortunately, current conventional medical practice contributes little to our understanding of how to keep a mother balanced and blissful during pregnancy, and even more importantly, after delivery, when her more active role of mothering begins. During the postpartum period, a mother often feels depleted and delicate, both physically and emotionally; yet she must face the added challenge of caring for her newborn while she struggles to recover her own strength.

Until now, knowledge of how to stay balanced and healthy during pregnancy has been fragmented and incomplete, while knowledge of how to recover after delivery has been missing entirely. Moreover, I have noticed in my own medical practice that women frequently date the onset of a chronic health condition to the birth of a child. This shows that pregnancy and delivery can cause fundamental imbalances that, if unchecked, can grow into serious health problems. These inadequacies in our current system point out the desperate need for new knowledge to help women meet the challenges of pregnancy and childbirth more successfully.

As a result of the exceptional work of Dr. Kumuda Reddy and her colleagues, Linda Egenes and Margaret Mullins, this need has now been met in this extraordinary and unique book for the expectant parent. *For a Blissful Baby* contains a wealth of knowledge from the oldest tradition of health care on earth—knowledge that will enable women to go through the physical and emotional transformations of childbirth and come out ahead, feeling on top of their lives, feeling better than ever before.

This knowledge is important not only for the health of the mother, but also for the health of her baby. For the mother is the main environment for her developing baby. Everything she eats or drinks, everything she thinks or feels, everything she sees or does has an immediate and intimate effect on her baby. Maharishi Vedic Medicine understands this profound connection and gives the mother the total knowledge she needs to create a balanced and nourishing environment for her growing baby.

This book addresses how to create a healthier, more contented, and more spiritually evolved baby through promoting balance in every area of life: physical, mental, behavioral, emotional, and spiritual. It covers everything from what foods to eat to what daily routine to follow to what kind of books, music, and other sensory experiences are best for both mother and child. Most importantly, it describes how the inner consciousness of the mother can be cultured to become the foundation for loving, compassionate, and giving behavior.

Every mother knows that the deepest connection between herself and her baby goes beyond anything physical, even beyond anything emotional. The deepest connection is on the level of consciousness itself. Consciousness is the deepest and most powerful level of life—the spiritual essence of life that connects everything to everything else.

Within consciousness are structured all the laws of nature that govern the physical universe. These laws of nature provide an exquisite blueprint for the baby and organize his or her development from the moment of conception on. If a mother develops her consciousness, then she enlivens natural law within her awareness, and this helps the whole process go more smoothly and more comfortably for both mother and child.

Through the development of consciousness, a mother balances the deepest level of her being. And when her deepest level is in balance, then everything unfolds in a more integrated and harmonious way. This book describes ways for a mother to develop her consciousness, very easily and effortlessly, even within a busy mom's routine.

In over twelve years of my own practice in Maharishi Vedic Medicine, I have seen this Consciousness-Based^SM approach benefit patients in dramatic ways. Women who have already had children, comment on the striking differences they notice when they follow a Vedic program in addition to their usual obstetric care. Instead of feeling emotionally fragile, tired, and overwhelmed after giving birth, they soon feel rejuvenated, revitalized, and balanced in both mind and body.

One of the most fulfilling experiences in my practice involved helping a young mother whose first child was conceived only with the use of fertility drugs, which she found very disturbing to her physical and emotional equilibrium. This unsettling period of infertility was followed by an uncomfortable pregnancy and a long, difficult labor. Furthermore, her newborn son developed serious health problems in the neonatal period, while she herself went through months of postpartum depression. Three years later, she came to me because she wanted another child, but wished to avoid the side effects of fertility drugs and the use of antidepressants postpartum, which could interfere with her ability to nurse her newborn.

Through the approaches of Maharishi Vedic Medicine, she first focused on regaining her own vibrant health and inner balance. On this solid foundation, she began to feel confident enough to attempt getting pregnant. Within a year, she conceived without the use of drugs, and gave birth to a baby girl who was healthy and indeed blissful. She herself experienced no depression after delivery, only increasing vitality and happiness. Moreover, when the new baby was only six months old, she handled her family's move to a foreign country with surprising comfort and ease.

Having children is a natural process. Women are designed to handle the awesome physical and emotional challenges involved. But it is essential for them to have proper knowledge and support before, during, and especially after the birth of their children.

Current medical practices have virtually nothing to offer the newly delivered mother. But with the therapies of Maharishi Vedic Medicine, the imbalances caused by the birth of a child are addressed and a mother recovers her strength quickly. This is important, because in order to give to her newborn, she must first be able to give.

If you are thinking about having a child—or are already counting the days!—this book will be your best friend on one of the most important and fulfilling journeys of your life.

Preface

The very thought of having a baby is accompanied by great expectations. It's a time filled with tenderness, love, and joy. Parents quite naturally want to do everything right for the sake of their special baby. My husband and I waited for five long years before we had our first child. I was doing my fellowship in anesthesiology at Mt. Sinai Hospital in New York City. It was a grueling schedule, but nonetheless we felt in our hearts it was the right time to have the baby. We spent our little free time planning for the birth with excitement, anticipation, and worry.

Early on we selected the best obstetrician and tried to do everything as properly as possible. I possessed all the latest medical knowledge and received expert care at a famous hospital, yet I knew something was missing. Something that I could not put my finger on—until I remembered the prenatal care that expectant mothers in my family had received while I was growing up in India. Pregnant women were showered with love and nurtured by the elder women in the home, and were given special foods and oil massages. Everyone in the household took care to keep the environment happy and positive so the new mother would always feel contented. Each of these caring actions seemed to have a special significance, although I did not understand it completely at the time.

The birth of my own baby and the postpartum period were both exhausting and painful. There was little help available to alleviate the pain and rejuvenate my body. My second pregnancy was an even greater challenge. A complicated pregnancy ended in premature delivery of beautiful twin girls. It took me months to recuperate. Even though I had the best possible medical treatment, I was painfully aware that I and every new mother needed something far beyond what conventional obstetric care could provide.

It was this realization that led me to Maharishi Vedic Medicine^SM, the Maharishi Vedic Approach to Health^SM, a few years later. This health care system has its roots in the timeless Vedic tradition of India, yet it is surprisingly modern in its approach to preventing and promoting health and well-being.

Once I learned about this practical health care system, I knew that this knowledge was profound and complete. Maharishi Vedic Medicine deals with all aspects of pregnancy, postpartum, and child care, and includes diet, behavior, exercise, rest, and stress reduction. It supplied the missing link—the intimate connection of mind and body with nature and the environment around us. And it provided the missing element of consciousness, which is the wholeness of life, the very basis of creation itself.

During each of my pregnancies, the nine months passed like a grand, eternal mystery sequentially unfolding itself. From the moment of conception all I could see in front of my eyes were the faces of blissful babies, whether in magazines, in crowds of people, in flowers, or in the twinkling stars at night. I remember my grandmother saying that every creation is a miracle, and that we have the ability to create all miracles with Mother Nature's support. I did not fully understand those words until I learned about Maharishi Vedic Medicine, which offers all the technologies to organize a healthy life with nature's support.

Now that I am using Maharishi Vedic Medicine in my practice, I enjoy seeing my patients grow in health and happiness as well. I find it truly heartening when my patients tell me how easy and happy their pregnancies are, and how different they feel during postpartum recovery now that they have this knowledge.

Most important of all, their babies are happier and healthier. They are a joy not only to the parents but to everyone who knows them. Growing up with the Maharishi Vedic Approach to Health is like sitting in the gentle lap of Mother Nature, where there is not only love and compassion, but an entire world of possibilities. It provides the path for health, happiness, and longevity for our babies. It has made possible a loving, friendly, and harmonious environment for our families. And because these children are not only loving and friendly to their parents, but also to the world, the Maharishi Vedic Approach to Health brings us the possibility of lasting peace. There is a new dawn on the horizon. Now is the time to reach out for this beautiful and practical knowledge.

I personally desire nothing less than healthy and harmonious families for all the blessed babies of the world. When I think of the womb and pregnancy, I am reminded of the *garbha* of traditional sacred temples in India. *Garbha* literally means "womb." It is the heart of the temple. It looks like a cave on the inside with a mountain projecting from the roof on the outside. It is as if the divine is reaching from the infinite, unmanifest field of life inside to the infinite, manifest universe on the outside. Or the inner self is reaching to the higher self. From the moment the construction of the garbha begins, the guardians of the temple proceed with many ceremonies to promote balance in the individual and the community and to enliven the transcendental, unbounded level of life.

People step into the garbha with multiple problems and stresses, but inside the garbha all experience that deep silence, joy, peace, and bliss. They become one with the divine. Everyone who steps into that environment experiences their own precious dignity as human beings. When they step out, the reality of the relative world returns, bringing with it the stress and strain of everyday life. But that moment in time is cherished forever and the desire to experience it again is strong.

Nature's womb in the mother is also such a sacred place. The natural technologies of Maharishi Vedic Medicine, especially the development of consciousness, create that most peaceful, harmonious, and nourishing environment for the baby to develop at all levels—mind, body, emotions, and spirit. The process of creating perfection in the physiology begins then, in the womb, and continues during the early years. Happiness, security, and self-esteem are cultivated in these babies' lives from their earliest days. And in the long run these natural procedures also improve health, immunity, and longevity.

We know that each child displays certain traits even at birth, which shape the individual personality and the course of life in general. Maharishi Vedic Medicine shows us that we can help every child reach his or her full potential, by enlivening health even from the moment of conception. We can become co-creators of the infinite miracle of having blissful babies and harmonious families. Now is the time to begin.

—Kumuda Reddy, M.D.

FOR A BLISSFUL BABY

PART I

A Healthy Pregnancy
for a Healthy Child

A Healthy Pregnancy for a Healthy Child

In most cultures, pregnancy is a time to be cherished, a time to nourish and protect yourself and your unborn child. The chapters in Part I describe Maharishi Vedic Medicine, also known as the Maharishi Vedic Approach to Health, which deeply nourishes mother and baby physically, mentally, emotionally, and spiritually through natural, effective treatments. As you read about this remarkably complete approach to mother and baby care—which covers everything from foods to fertility to the effects of sound on the fetus—you will feel comforted and secure that it contains the knowledge to help give your child the best possible start.

In Chapter One you will learn about the many facets of this system of health care, and how its natural therapies nourish mother and child throughout pregnancy, delivery, and postpartum. Chapter Two describes the unique role of the cornerstone technique of the Maharishi Vedic Approach to Health—the Transcendental Meditation® program. By removing stress and providing deep rest, this simple, effortless technique can help you stay free of fatigue and anxiety throughout the challenges of giving birth. Chapter Three identifies the three physiological and psychological principles that link your nature with nature around you. It explains how these three principles can be kept in balance for a healthy pregnancy.

In Chapter Four, we discuss the major influences on fertility and describe natural methods to improve your own health to conceive a healthier baby. The various stages of development of the fetus are discussed in Chapter Five. Chapter Six goes deeply into principles for healthy eating during pregnancy, and describes how to improve your digestion. Chapter Seven identifies the basic rhythms of nature, and tells how to structure your daily routine to bring yourself in tune with natural cycles and feel more energetic while you are pregnant.

Maharishi Vedic Medicine recognizes that it is essential for the mother to be happy in order to produce a contented, healthy baby. This is such an important area that we've devoted Chapter Eight to staying happy during pregnancy.

"Maharishi's Vedic Approach to Health offers to reestablish balance between the body and its own inner intelligence through Vedic Knowledge and its application."   —Maharishi Mahesh Yogi[1]

"The means to achieve Vedic Health is to develop Vedic Consciousness—fully awakened, fully enlightened consciousness."

—Maharishi Mahesh Yogi[2]

CHAPTER ONE

A Complete Approach to Pregnancy and Postpartum

Congratulations. You're having a baby. You're about to start on the most important adventure of your life, a journey that will put you in touch with an essential creative process—giving birth to a new human being.

If this is your first child, chances are you're a little nervous, a little apprehensive that you are responsible for the well-being of your child. You probably have a thousand questions about the care and nurturing of your new baby. And even if this isn't your first child, you probably want to know how to be better prepared for everything this time around.

In these pages you'll find a whole new way of looking at human life—from conception through the first year. This book unfolds principles of healthy living during pregnancy and the critical few weeks after giving birth, and helps you care for your newborn. It gives a glimpse into the eternal continuum of life that you and your children are all part of. And it tells you how to give your baby the best possible start in life.

What is *Maharishi Vedic Medicine*?

This book offers a total approach to mother and baby care, based on Maharishi Vedic Medicine. This is the most comprehensive and complete system of health care imaginable—covering the full range of life, from the spiritual, mental, emotional, physical, and behavioral health of the individual to the health of the environment and the society as a whole. Also called the Maharishi Vedic Approach to Health, it takes into account your whole self— how the things you feel, think, say, breathe, touch, smell, hear, and do affect the health and well-being of both you and your baby. No part of life is left out of the Maharishi Vedic Approach to Health. It always amazes me* how all-encompassing this age-old system of medicine is, and how effective it is in treating the needs of my modern patients.

Veda means knowledge. Maharishi Vedic Medicine is based on the knowledge of the Veda and Vedic Literature, the oldest record of human experience, which contains the complete knowledge of natural law and of the specific laws of nature that govern all of life and living throughout the universe. The Vedic tradition has given us the oldest system of health care in the world, originally cognized by the great seers, or "Maharishis," of the ancient Vedic civilization in India. While it has been in continuous use since then, the ravages of wars, foreign domination, and simply the passage of time have taken their toll on the purity, the practices, and the full understanding of this approach to health care. Unfortunately in recent centuries its foundation in the development of consciousness became hidden from view. What remained was chiefly herbal remedies (many of whose original formulas had been lost) drawn from the *Ayurvedic* tradition. *Ayur-Veda* (literally "the science of life span") draws on knowledge from several aspects of Vedic Literature which could broadly be classified as "medical." Two ancient sages who contributed a great deal to the Ayurvedic tradition were named Charaka and Sushruta. They are responsible for much of the information

---

* Although there are three authors, at times you'll find "I" or "me" used when Dr. Kumuda Reddy is speaking from her clinical experience.

contained in this present book, and their texts, named respectively the *Charaka Samhita* and the *Sushruta Samhita,* are referred to frequently in the coming pages.

Maharishi Mahesh Yogi, who is the founder of the Transcendental Meditation program, is responsible for resuscitating Ayur-Veda in the twentieth century. Gathering together the greatest living Ayurvedic experts, delving deep into the classical texts, Maharishi supervised his Council of *Vaidyas* as they restored the purity of Ayur-Veda, including its true basis, the development of consciousness. The resulting system of "complete" Ayur-Veda, now called the *Maharishi Ayur-Veda®* program, combines a profound theoretical understanding of both ancient and modern medicine with a great body of scientific research on its effectiveness.

Maharishi Vedic Medicine is broader still. It draws not just on the Ayurvedic texts but on all forty major values of natural law contained in the Veda and Vedic Literature to help the individual to bring mind, body, and environment into a comprehensive state of balance. Creating higher states of consciousness and a state of lasting health and happiness may seem like an unattainable goal, yet thousands of people throughout the world are learning what it is like to live without disease, suffering, or unhappiness through this approach. In this book we'll show you both research and personal reports which attest to this.

What sets Maharishi Vedic Medicine apart from other health care systems is that it takes into account the full range of natural law, and that it focuses first on *developing the consciousness of the individual.* You probably have heard that the majority of diseases are psychosomatic, meaning that even though the symptoms appear in the physical body, the disease is caused or aggravated by mental or emotional imbalances. Maharishi Vedic Medicine starts by helping the individual to enliven the inner intelligence of the body, expand the awareness, and remove mental, emotional and physical stress. On that basis, the other approaches of treating the body, emotions, behavior, and environment are much more effective.

What *Maharishi Vedic Medicine* Offers Mothers and Babies

Maharishi Vedic Medicine focuses on creating balance on three levels—for the mother, for the baby, and in the relationship between them. It accomplishes this through stress-reduction techniques, diet, special Vedic massage procedures, rejuvenation programs, and many other valuable recommendations.

This book gives special attention to one of the most critical problems for new mothers—postpartum fatigue. Giving birth is one of the greatest challenges that a woman will ever face. While the mother's heart is totally enlivened with love for her new baby, her body is under demands never faced before. She needs to balance and strengthen her body and emotions so she can give her baby nourishment and love.

Maharishi Vedic Medicine fills a gap in modern obstetrics, which emphasizes only the areas of pregnancy, labor, and delivery. It provides a fundamentally different kind of knowledge to create ideal health in the mother and baby at conception, throughout pregnancy, and during postpartum—the delicate first few weeks after birth.

It is one of the greatest joys of my practice to recommend the Maharishi Vedic Approach to Health to new mothers. They report that their babies are healthier, with less colic, digestive problems, and early childhood sickness. Even more importantly, these mothers find that they can recover much more quickly from the fatigue of pregnancy and delivery, and can devote more love and attention to their children. Very naturally, by taking care to maintain her own health, the mother directly helps her baby.

The Maharishi Vedic Approach to Health enriches the tender bonds of love and nourishment that naturally exist between parents and their children. In fact, it offers programs to help structure more ideal health for the whole family, making the adventure of raising children much more fulfilling.

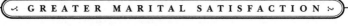

GREATER MARITAL SATISFACTION

Higher Marital Adjustment in *TM* Program Meditators

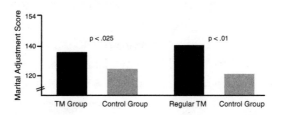

Married women who had learned the Transcendental Meditation program showed greater marital satisfaction than matched non-meditating controls. Those practicing the TM technique on a regular basis showed an even stronger effect.

Reference: E.N. Aron and A. Aron, "Transcendental Meditation Program and Marital Adjustment," *Psychological Reports*, 51 (1982), pp. 887-890.

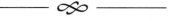

Reduced Family Problems

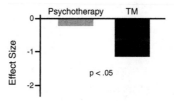

A group of Vietnam veterans was randomly assigned either to practice the Transcendental Meditation technique or to participate in psychotherapy. Those who learned the Transcendental Meditation technique improved significantly on eight psychological measures, including a reduction in family problems, while the psychotherapy participants showed no significant improvement over the same three-month period. This study indicates the TM program dissolves deep-rooted stress and develops a more relaxed individual who can recover from stressful experiences more quickly.

Reference: J.S. Brooks and T. Scarano, "Transcendental Meditation in the Treatment of Post-Vietnam Adjustment," *Journal of Counseling and Development*, 64 (1986), pp. 212-215.

Mothers Report the Benefits

In working with mothers who follow the Maharishi Vedic Approach to Health during pregnancy and postpartum, I notice that they recover very rapidly, lose their excess weight quickly and easily, and have much more energy to nurture and care for their babies. I am extremely impressed because I have never seen an instance of postpartum depression among these mothers. Mothers look healthier, more rested, and happier.

Mary was one such mother. With her first child, she had not yet heard of Maharishi Vedic Medicine. She recalls, *"I gained a tremendous amount of weight, had a fairly easy delivery, and was completely overwhelmed by the responsibilities of becoming a new mother. Changing from a career woman to a mother was quite an adjustment. I remember calling up my friend and saying, 'Please come over and rescue me. I can't even get up and go to the bathroom. Every time I move, he screams!'*

"Obviously, I coped, and since I had cared for my younger brothers and sisters it was easy for me to figure out how to care for him. But the fatigue really knocked me out, which was what made it so difficult. It took me months to recover, and longer to lose the excess weight."

With her second child, Mary was able to use Maharishi Vedic Medicine as complementary care for her pregnancy. Following the birth, she received a complete program of daily massage from a trained technician who visited her home daily for six weeks, a special diet to help her digestion get back to normal, and herbal supplements.

"One of the most amazing experiences I ever had was my first massage after giving birth. It was so blissful and such an amazing contrast from what my body had gone through to deliver. It was so completely nourishing. I felt so much more able to give love to my baby. It made me feel like a queen (and it's the only thing that could at that point in time). Before the massage I felt big and heavy, and every muscle in me was sore—but after the massage I thought, 'Oh, I feel so good.'"

"I realized that nourishing the new mother is so important because not only are you very, very tired and have a new baby to care for who wants you almost every moment, but you have your husband and the rest of the family to care for, too. It's an incredible challenge, but the massage and diet and the whole program just restores you. You're looking for that balance in activity—of feeling content and not feeling overwhelmed. With the recommendations from Maharishi Vedic Medicine, I was able to achieve that balance. With my second birth, I recovered from fatigue in just six weeks, and lost my excess weight, too."

Another mother reported that by following this system, she was able to avoid digestive problems, and felt energetic and fatigue-free throughout her pregnancy. Other mothers report that the infant massage (described in Chapter Fourteen) gives them an additional opportunity to bond with their babies, and helps the children build immunity and suffer less colic and gas.

Throughout this book you will be meeting many of these mothers—mothers who are living the beautiful principles of the Maharishi Vedic Approach to Health, and giving their babies a gentle and strong start in life.

The *Maharishi Ayur-Veda* Program for You and Your Child

There are many approaches coming from the Maharishi Ayur-Veda healthcare program that help improve the well-being of mother and child. The Maharishi Ayur-Veda program forms the basis for much of the material presented in this book. As was mentioned earlier, Ayur-Veda is an important aspect of Veda and Vedic Literature that focuses on medicine—preventing disease, promoting ideal health, and lengthening lifespan—and helping to bring individual and collective life into harmony with natural law.

Because health care starts with conception, the Maharishi Ayur-Veda program for mothers gives in-depth knowledge for healthy conception, pregnancy, delivery, postpartum care, and children's health. Here are some areas of Maharishi Ayur-Veda health care that are particularly valuable for new mothers. These appear in greater detail in later chapters:

Maharishi Rejuvenation^{SM} *Therapy:* This includes natural, seasonal procedures (called *panchakarma*) to eliminate accumulated stresses and cleanse the body of residual toxins through a combination of massage therapies, gentle heat treatments, eliminative procedures, and ways to restore balance in biological rhythms. The herbalized oil massage therapies have special importance in relaxing and rejuvenating the body during the postpartum period, when every cell has been depleted by the exertion of giving birth.

One research study showed that people who followed the recommendations of Maharishi Vedic Medicine enjoyed improved general health, digestion, elimination, sleep, energy levels, and resistance to illness. At the same time, they experienced less worry, depression, and emotional disturbance.

Dietary Recommendations: The food you eat while you're pregnant will directly influence your baby's health. And after you give birth, your diet is equally important in creating wholesome breast milk and restoring needed energy. The science of eating the right foods at the right time is a major area of the Maharishi Ayur-Veda program, and includes specific dietary guidelines for pregnancy and postpartum.

Herbal Preparations: One of the Maharishi Ayur-Veda program's great contributions has been the rediscovery of detailed instructions for preparing a large number of plant and mineral compounds to prevent and treat disorders. Many of these are also helpful in nourishing the new mother and baby. Special herbal preparations called *rasayanas* revitalize the body, improve mental functioning, promote long life, and enhance the development of consciousness. Research has shown that they have a wide-ranging effect, from increasing intelligence[3] to enhancing immunity.[4] Traditionally, these are an important part of prenatal and postpartum care.

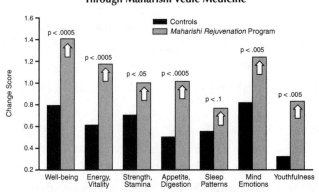

⸲ MAHARISHI REJUVENATION THERAPY ⸲

**Physiological and Psychological Improvements
Through Maharishi Vedic Medicine**

This study found that people who participated in a one-week Maharishi Rejuvenation℠ program of the Maharishi Vedic Approach to Health improved significantly across a wide range of measures. Control subjects who received only intellectual knowledge of this program and its principles for the same amount of time did not show the same amount of improvement. These findings indicate that the Maharishi Rejuvenation program, which is recommended to be applied seasonally to remove accumulated physiological toxins of the season, promotes physiological and psychological balance.

Another study, published in a German medical journal, examined various physiological and psychological changes that occurred in subjects participating in a two-week Maharishi Rejuvenation program. Improvements included reduced cholesterol and urea, reduced bodily complaints and strains, reduced irritability and psychological inhibition, and greater stability and openness.

References: 1. R.H. Schneider, K.L. Cavanaugh, H.S. Kasture, S. Rothenberg, R. Averbach, D. Robinson, And R.K. Wallace, "Health Promotion with a Traditional System of Natural Health Care: Maharishi Ayur-Veda," *Journal of Social Behavior and Personality*, 5 (3) (1990), pp. 1-27

2. R. Waldschutz, "Influence of Maharishi Ayur-Veda Purification Treatment on Physiological and Psychological Health," *Erfahrungsheilkunde-Acta Medica Empirica*, 11 (1988), pp. 720-729.

Daily Routine in Tune with Nature's Rhythms: The daily and seasonal rhythms of the sun have a great effect on your health. The program for mothers provided by Maharishi Ayur-Veda health care includes an entire area of recommendations to help bring your body's daily and seasonal cycles in tune with nature's cycles, so that you and your baby can enjoy greater health and happiness every day and throughout the year.

Approach through the Senses: Hearing, touch, sight, taste, and smell can be used to balance your mind and body. The Maharishi Ayur-Veda program includes therapies to enliven each of the senses (e.g., aromatherapy) and correct imbalances throughout the mind and body.

In this chapter, you have already learned many new terms and concepts. Yet this is not a complicated book, and is by design easy to read and accessible to busy mothers-to-be.

It is important to note, as you read this book, that Maharishi Vedic Medicine does not in any way replace or preclude the advice of your primary care obstetrician. The beauty of Maharishi Vedic Medicine is that it complements modern medical care— filling in the gaps and enhancing quality of life in a simple, natural way that does not conflict with standard medical care. In my practice, I use both systems of medicine to their best advantage.

In any case, this book is not intended to give medical advice, since you need to consult a physician to be diagnosed and treated for your individual health needs. Rather, this book offers a vision of possibilities, a new paradigm of health and happiness for mothers and children of the world.

New Approaches to Nourish Mother and Baby

Maharishi Vedic Medicine addresses the whole range of natural law, applying knowledge not only from the Ayurvedic texts but from all forty branches of the Veda and Vedic Literature. Much of this knowledge is missing from modern medicine today. The following are five of the most fundamental aspects of the Maharishi Vedic Medicine.

1. Consciousness: Today physicians everywhere understand the correlation between stress and health. At no time is it more important for you to be relaxed and rested than when you are carrying a baby. The Transcendental Meditation program has been scientifically proven to be the most effective method available to reduce stress. Research also indicates that people who practice the Transcendental Meditation program experience improvement in many areas of life: physical and mental health, emotional balance, mental ability, social relationships, job performance, and family life. I have seen my own patients clear up a wide range of mental and physical ailments just by practicing this simple technique twice a day. And the mothers I see who practice the Transcendental Meditation are freer from fatigue and enjoy their pregnancies and mothering experience more.

2. **Collective Health Care:** As a mother you are concerned about the world your child grows up in. How can you prevent natural and man-made disasters from affecting your children? Crime, war, tension in society, environmental toxins and pollutants— all of these are societal problems which may have a direct influence on the health of your family.

   The collective approach to health, which includes large groups of people practicing the Transcendental Meditation program (and the more advanced practice called the TM-Sidhi® program), can help balance collective consciousness, eliminate tension and stress in the community, and nation—and create a healthier world.

3. **Pulse Diagnosis:** By using a particular method of pulse reading, a physician trained in Maharishi Vedic Medicine can detect current and future imbalances and determine the healthiest diet, daily and seasonal routines, and herbal supplements for your specific mind-body system. Pulse diagnosis is an extremely effective diagnostic tool, because it can help the physician detect imbalances *before* they develop into full-blown symptoms. Traditionally it is used as part of primary care for moth-

---

⋌ C O L L E C T I V E   H E A L T H   C A R E ⋋

Maharishi Effect: Improved Quality of Life and Reduced Conflict in the Middle East Through Group Practice of the *Transcendental Meditation* and *TM-Sidhi* Programs

This study indicates that group practice of the Maharishi Transcendental Medita-

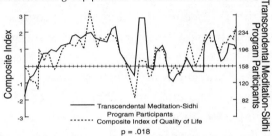

tion and TM-Sidhi programs improved the quality of life in Israel as measured by improvements on an index consisting of reduced crime rate, reduced traffic accidents, reduced fires, the reduced number of war deaths in Lebanon, increases in the national stock market, and improvements in national mood. The chart above shows the strong correpondence between the number of TM-Sidhi program participants in the group in Jerusalem and a composite index of all the above variables.

References: 1. D.W. Orme-Johnson, C.N. Alexander, J.L. Davies, H.M. Chandler, and W.E. Larimore, "International Peace Project in the Middle East: The Effects of the Maharishi Technology of the Unified Field," *Journal of Conflict Resolution*, 32 (4) (1988), pp. 776-812.

2. J.L. Davies and C.N. Alexander, "Alleviating Political Violence Through Enhancing Coherence in Collective Consciousness: Impact Assessment Analyses of the Lebanon Wars," *Dissertation Abstracts International*, 49 (8) (1988), p. 2381A.

---

ers and babies. The process of pulse diagnosis itself helps bring the body back into balance, and therefore in that sense also is a powerful tool for prevention.

4. **The Effect of the Near Environment on Health:** You may not realize that one of the most important influences on your health is found in the buildings you live in and work in. According to the Maharishi Vedic Approach to Health, a number of diseases arise just from the structure of these buildings. The knowledge of building in accord with natural law is included in one of the

forty aspects of the Maharishi Vedic Approach to Health, called Maharishi Sthapatya Veda® design. People who live and work in buildings that are designed to be in harmony with the laws of nature find that nature protects and promotes their success in every area of life, including health.

If the home is not designed properly, the behavior, thinking, and speech of the family members will be out of tune with natural law, creating problems and obstacles to good fortune, good health, and family harmony. Maharishi Sthapatya Veda design explains how to design a building with correct orientation, direction, and proportion to promote only good influences from the environment. This may appear to be an abstract level of consideration in the field of health care, but the benefits are very practical. People who live and work in buildings designed according to these principles find that they think more clearly, are less tired, feel happier and healthier, and experience greater business success.

5. **The Effect of the Distant Environment on Health:** It is well known that the sun and moon have an effect on health. As the earth rotates on its axis, we experience the cycles of night and day; as it revolves around the sun, we experience the changes of seasons. These daily and seasonal rhythms affect our moods, our hormones, and our general state of health and well-being. The moon also has a known effect on human behavior and internal cycles of the body. Maharishi Vedic Medicine takes these influences into account, as well as the influence of the distant planets and stars.

These distant planets and stars are our "cosmic counterparts." What does this mean? Simply that our consciousness, our DNA, our own body, are all expressions of the same fundamental structures of nature's intelligence that are found expressed in the entire universe. The planets and stars have their exact counterparts in the human physiology, and thus there is a profound connectedness between the individual and the universe, be-

Forty Approaches are Forty Aspects of Natural Law, as Contained in the Veda and Vedic Literature

In describing the Maharishi Vedic Approach to Health, sometimes various branches of the Vedic Literature are mentioned. For example, the Maharishi Vedic Astrology program comes from the knowledge of the aspect of the Vedic Literature called *Jyotish*, and Maharishi Sthapatya Veda design comes from the aspect called *Sthapatya Veda*.

There are forty aspects of the Vedic Literature; together, they express the knowledge of all the fundamental structures of natural law in the entire universe. Maharishi Vedic Medicine offers knowledge drawn from all forty aspects of the Vedic Literature—because they apply to health and well-being in every area of human life.

Based on Maharishi's insights into the Veda and Vedic Literature, Professor Tony Nader, M.D., Ph.D., an MIT-trained neuroscientist, has recently discovered that the different aspects of the human physiology form an exact replica of the patterns of intelligence that are expressed in the forty aspects of the Veda and Vedic Literature. This discovery reveals that the inner intelligence of the body, which governs all functions in the human physiology, is in actuality the same laws of nature that govern the entire universe. There is a saying from the Vedic Literature that expresses this idea in a simple way. It says, "As is the individual, so is the universe. As is the microcosm, so is the macrocosm."[5]

This recognition—that the total range of natural law that constitutes the Veda is the same natural law expressed in our human consciousness, mind, and body—helps modern science to bridge the gap between mind and body, between consciousness and physiology, and between the individual, the environment, and the universe. And even more importantly, this knowledge demonstrates that it is possible to treat the body completely from the level of the total intelligence of natural law. In other words, if we enliven the total potential of natural law at the basis of the physiology, the whole body can be transformed. If we awaken nature's intelligence in the body, we can create ideal health.

tween the individual body and the cosmic body. These cosmic counterparts have a direct influence on the mind, body, behavior, and environment day after day, year after year, season after season. To maintain perfect health, it is important to know what influences are coming to you, so you can take steps to neutralize the negative ones and to enhance the positive ones.

The Maharishi Vedic Astrology^SM program contains the knowledge of the cycles of time, explaining how our cosmic counterparts are an intimate part of all changes and developments in life and of how life unfolds sequentially from the moment of birth. The Maharishi Vedic Astrology program analyzes these mathematical cycles to predict future trends in health, fortune, and all other areas of life.

The Maharishi Vedic Astrology program is especially helpful in planning the conception and birth of a child. If the timing is favorable, everything will go more smoothly and bring more joy and happiness to the parents and child. If obstacles are foreseen at the anticipated time of conception or birth, the parents may be advised to wait until a better time to conceive, or may be advised to take advantage of the corrective measures offered by the Maharishi Yagya^SM program. These include performances to mitigate any negative influences that could cloud the health or good fortune of the family. The goal of the Maharishi Yagya program is to "avert the danger that has not yet come," and through these procedures can help to bring the body and mind back into balance.

Summary

Maharishi Vedic Medicine, the Maharishi Vedic Approach to Health, contains a complete program that naturally promotes healthy pregnancy, recovery from postpartum fatigue, and happy babies. This complete program, which includes the Transcendental

Meditation program, a special massage for mother and baby, specific dietary recommendations, herbal supplements, and many other therapies, fills a gap in modern obstetrics, which offers only partial support to postpartum mothers.

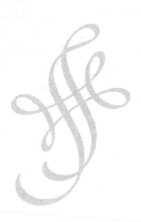

"A perfectly healthy person lives in the state of enlightenment, with the natural ability to spontaneously use the total organizing power of Natural Law to accomplish any goal without strain."
—Maharishi Mahesh Yogi[6]

"Diseases do not afflict an individual who is endowed with excellence of thoughts, speech and acts which are ultimately blissful, independent thinking, clear understanding, knowledge, observance of spiritual prescriptions and love for meditation."
—*Charaka Samhita*[7]

CHAPTER TWO

Developing Consciousness to Give Your Baby the Best Possible Start in Life

As you prepare for your baby's conception and birth, chances are you are thinking about the miracle of life itself. If you are like most mothers, you are in awe of your body's ability to create new life in your womb. Without your conscious effort or knowledge, billions of cells shape themselves into the human being who will become your son or daughter.

And you probably wonder how to give your baby the very best start in life. Will you know how to care for him or her during your pregnancy and in the tender first weeks after birth? And what should you eat and what should you do to stay healthy?

These are all natural concerns of a loving mother-to-be. This book will help answer these concerns, but for your baby to be truly healthy and happy, the most important thing you can do is *relax and enjoy the entire process, and allow your body's natural intelligence to effortlessly nourish you and your baby.* After all, it is this intelligence that orchestrates and coordinates the infinite number of cells, organs, and working parts of your body; it is this same intelligence that keeps the planets orbiting the sun in perfect synchrony. And it is this intelligence that creates a very perfect human being from its start as a single cell in your womb.

In fact, enlivening this powerful intelligence of nature within you is the most important aim of Maharishi Vedic Medicine. All of the therapies and treatments attempt to wake up your inner healing intelligence, to balance and strengthen your body from within.

I was trained in conventional medicine to think of the body as a machine, with thousands of individual parts that have to be treated in isolation. In reality, it is just the opposite—the body is a manifestation of this inner intelligence of natural law. This inner intelligence is also understood in Maharishi Vedic Medicine to be a field of pure consciousness—and is open to direct experience at the deepest level of the mind. If you enliven this inner intelligence from the deepest level of consciousness, you can affect the health and well-being of your entire body, mind, and emotions in one stroke, just as watering the root of a tree nourishes all of the branches and leaves.

That is why one of the first things I prescribe to my patients when they tell me they want to conceive a baby is the Transcendental Meditation technique. Although all of the therapies and recommendations of Maharishi Vedic Medicine aim to enliven consciousness, this technique is the most powerful and is therefore the cornerstone treatment. Because it allows the individual to directly experience and enliven pure consciousness, the Transcendental Meditation technique can have a deeply transforming effect on the physical, mental, emotional, and spiritual health of both you and your child.

Benefits for You and Your Baby

The Transcendental Meditation program was founded by Maharishi Mahesh Yogi, and it comes from an age-old succession of masters from the Vedic tradition of knowledge.

When Maharishi first came to America in 1959, he invited research scientists to study the physiological effects of this simple technique. At that time it was considered a radical idea that the mind and body are connected. The first scientific research, published in *Science* in 1970, showed that during the practice of the Transcendental Meditation technique the mind becomes more awake and the body becomes deeply rested.[8] Today more than 600 research studies have been conducted in 200 research institutions and universities in 30 countries around the world on the benefits of this unique state of "restful alertness." They show a wide range of improvements in mental, physical, emotional, spiritual, and even environmental health.

Research shows that the Transcendental Meditation technique **reduces—**

- mental and physical stress
- medical care usage and hospitalization by 50 percent
- systolic blood pressure
- high cholesterol
- infectious disease
- anxiety
- tension
- depression
- use of caffeine, tobacco, alcohol, and prescribed and non-prescribed drugs

Research also shows that it **improves—**

- clarity of thinking
- energy levels
- mind-body coordination
- intuition
- happiness
- harmonious relationships at home and at work.

You can imagine how all of these benefits can help you become

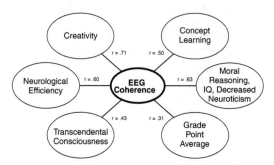

⌖ IMPROVED MENTAL HEALTH ⌖

Optimization of Brain Functioning

Higher levels of EEG coherence measured during the practice of the Trancendental Meditation technique are significantly correlated with increased fluency of verbal creativity, increased efficiency in learning new concepts, more principled moral reasoning, higher verbal IQ, decreased neuroticism, higher academic achievement, clearer experiences of Transcendental Consciousness, and increased neurological efficiency, as measured by faster recovery of the H-reflex.

References: The chart above was constructed with data from the following four studies:
1. D.W. Orme-Johnson and C.T. Haynes, "EEG Phase Coherence, Pure Consciousness, Creativity, and TM-Sidhi Experiences," *International Journal of Neuroscience,* 13 (1981), pp. 211–217.
2. M.C. Dillbek, D.W. Orme-Johnson, and R.K. Wallace, "Frontal EEG Coherence, H-Reflex Recovery, Concept Learning, and the TM-Sidhi Program," *International Journal of Neuroscience,* 15 (1981), pp. 151–157.
3. C.T. Haynes, J.R. Hebert, W. Reber, and D.W. Orme-Johnson, "Psychophysiology of Advanced Participants in the Transcendental Meditation Program: Correlations of EEG Coherence, Creativity, H-Reflex Recovery, and Experiences of Transcendental Consciousness," *Scientific Research on the* Transcendental Meditation *Program: Collected Papers, Volume I* (1977), pp. 208–212.
4. D.W. Orme-Johnson, "Factor Analysis of EEG Coherence Parameters," *Scientific Research on the* Transcendental Meditation *and* TM-Sidhi *Program: Collected Papers, Volume 4* (1989), pp. 2245–2266.

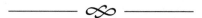

More Positive Self-Image

Subjects experienced an improved self-concept one month after starting the Transcendental Meditation program. Subjects found that their perception of their "actual self" became closer to their "ideal self," and they also developed a more strongly defined concept of their "actual self." No similar changes were observed for matched controls.

Reference: M.J. Turnbull and H. Norris, "Effects of Transcendental Meditation on Self-Identity Indices and Personality," *British Journal of Psychology,* 73 (1982), pp. 57-68.

⸱⸱ I M P R O V E D   P H Y S I C A L   H E A L T H ⸱⸱

Reduced Hospitalization and Doctor's Visits

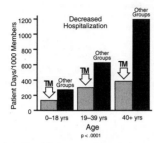 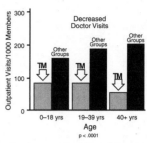

A study of health insurance statistics over a five-year period found that 2000 participants in the Transcendental Meditation program had less than half the doctor visits and hospitalization than other groups of comparable age, gender, profession, and insurance terms. The difference between the groups was greatest for individuals over 40. In addition, the TM program practitioners had markedly fewer incidents of illness in 17 medical treatment categories.

References: 1. D.W. Orme-Johnson, "Medical Care Utilization and the Transcendental Meditation Program," *Psychosomatic Medicine*, 49 (1) (1987), pp. 493-507.
2. D.W. Orme-Johnson and R. Schneider, "Reduced Health Care Utilization in Transcendental Meditation Practitioners," presented at the conference of the Society for Behavioral Medicine (Washington, D.C.), March 22, 1987.

∞

Decreased Stress Hormone

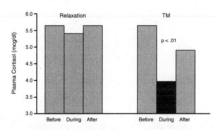

Cortisol is a hormone in the bloodstream which is found in large concentrations during stress, fasting, or dehydration. This study found that people who had been practicing the Transcendental Meditation program for three to five years had significantly lower cortisol levels during the TM technique compared to just before beginning the technique, and significantly lower levels during meditation compared to controls who were resting with eyes closed.

References: 1. R. Jevning, A.F. Wilson, and J.M. Davidson, "Adrenocortical Activity During Meditation," *Hormones and Behavior*, 10 (1978), pp. 54-60.
2. A.J.W. Bevan, R.G. Symons, C.G. Beng, M.L. Wellby, "Short-term Endocrine Changes in Transcendental Meditation," *Proceedings of the Endocrine Society of Australia*, 2 (1979), Abstract 56.

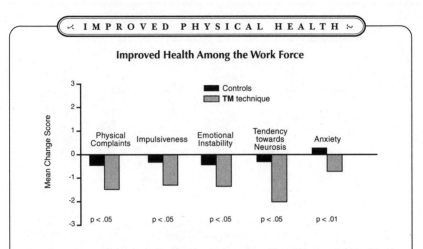

In a large 5-month study period by the National Institute of Industrial Health of the Japanese Ministry of Labor and the St. Marianna Medical Institution, 447 industrial workers of Sumitomo Heavy Industries were taught the Transcendental Meditation technique and compared to 321 workers who did not learn it. The Transcendental Meditation technique group showed significant decreases in health problems.

References: 1. T. Haratani and T. Henmi, "Effects of Transcendental Meditation (TM) on the Mental Health of Industrial Workers," *Japanese Journal of Industrial Health,* 32 (1990), p. 346.
2. T. Haratani and T. Henmi, "Effects of Transcendental Meditation (TM) on the Health Behavior of Industrial Workers," *Japanese Journal of Public Health,* 37 (1990), p. 729.

a better mother, because the best way to prepare for motherhood is to be as healthy, happy, and rested as you can.

How It Works

The best thing about the Transcendental Meditation technique is that it doesn't take a lot of time—just twenty minutes twice a day. My patients who practice it regularly find that they have more energy and efficiency, which more than makes up for the time spent.

You practice the technique sitting comfortably with your eyes closed. It is completely easy and effortless. Unlike other meditation procedures you may have heard of, it does not involve any concentration. For this reason it is completely natural—you are never straining against your mind. And it does not involve any religion or philosophy. I have recommended it to patients of all different cultures, religions, and nationalities.

During the Transcendental Meditation technique, the mind settles down to quieter and quieter levels of activity, "transcending" the surface level of thinking. As your mind settles down and reaches its simplest state of awareness, it begins to experience the field of infinite intelligence, energy, and bliss inside you. This completely self-referral state of awareness is called "pure consciousness." Gaining familiarity with this field of pure consciousness every day helps you begin to unfold your full potential in life. Many of my patients report that they start feeling in tune with nature.

When the mind settles down, it has a corresponding effect on your body, providing a deep state of rest. This is especially vital for pregnancy and postpartum—because it allows you to receive a quality of rest that is more effective than that found in sleep. And it allows deeper stresses to dissolve and fade away, clearing the way to better health and improved resistance to disease.[9]

Many people who practice this remarkable technique find themselves developing in many ways, becoming more the person they want to be. It is really the birthright of every person to live a life in freedom—freedom from disease, from worry, from problems in life. This is what the Vedic texts describe as the state of enlightenment, a state of perfect health and balance in life. This is the vision that Maharishi Vedic Medicine offers to each of us and to our children.

A Story About Consciousness

Sometimes discussing the field of consciousness that is experienced through practicing the Transcendental Meditation technique can sound very abstract. I would like to share one of my favorite stories from my home country, because it made my own understanding clearer. It is from a branch of the Vedic Literature called the Upanishads, which are known for their illuminating expressions of the universal Self, the ocean of pure knowledge, power, and bliss found inside everyone. It is the story of Shvetaketu (pronounced Shvay'-tuh-kay-too), a boy who learned an important lesson from his father.

The Story of Shvetaketu
(from the *Chhandogya Upanishad*)[10]

Many years ago in a village in India there lived a boy named Shvetaketu. Shvetaketu was the son of a great and wise man, Uddalaka.

When Shvetaketu turned twelve, his father said to him, "My dear son, follow the tradition of our family and become a man of knowledge." And so, as was the custom then, Shvetaketu went to the home of his teacher to study.

After many years, he finished his studies and returned to his father's house. His father noticed that something was different about his son Shvetaketu. Shvetaketu thought he knew everything there was to know.

Shvetaketu's father saw his son's pride. "My dear son," he asked, "I wonder if you have learned the wisdom of the Veda. Can you hear what cannot be heard by the ear? Can you see what cannot be seen by the eyes? Do you know what cannot be known by the mind?"

"What do you mean, dear Father?" asked Shvetaketu in surprise.

"Do you know that by knowing which everything else becomes known?" asked his father.

"What is this teaching, Father?" asked Shvetaketu.

"My son, when you know one lump of clay, you know all that is made of clay.

"When you know one nugget of gold, you know all that is made of gold.

"When you know one pair of iron tongs, you know all that is made of iron."

"I have not yet learned this teaching," said Shvetaketu humbly. "Please, Father, teach me."

"As you wish, my dear son," said his father.

"In the beginning there was an unbounded ocean of consciousness, one without a second. The ocean of Being thought to itself, 'I am one—may I be many,' and created light. Light thought to itself, 'I am one—may I be many,' and created water. Water thought to itself, 'I am one—may I be many,' and created matter.

"One unbounded ocean of consciousness became light, water, and matter. And the three became many. In this way the whole universe was created as an unbounded ocean of consciousness ever unfolding within itself.

"That infinite source of the whole universe, the Self of all that is, the ocean of pure consciousness, that essence of all things— that is truth. That is the unbounded Self. Of that you are created. That thou art, Shvetaketu."

"Please, honored Sir, tell me more of this teaching," said Shvetaketu.

"As you wish, my dear son," said his father. "Come with me to the orchard."

When they arrived at the orchard, he said, "See the bees collecting nectar? Once the nectar is gathered, it does not say, 'I am the essence of the apple blossom,' or 'I am the essence of the orange blossom.' No, the nectar joins with itself, and is called honey.

"In the same way, Shvetaketu, when people contact the ocean of pure consciousness, they become one with it and do not remember their individual natures. Yet when they are active, they again become a teacher, a farmer, or a goldsmith.

"That subtle essence of the whole world, the Self of all that is, the ocean of pure consciousness—that is truth. That is the eternal Self. Of that you are created. That thou art, Shvetaketu."

"Please, honored sir, teach me more," Shvetaketu said.

"As you wish, my dear. Come with me to the river."

When they arrived at the river, they stood at its banks and watched the water rushing by. His father said, "As the rivers flow to the east and merge with the sea, they become the sea itself. Once they are the sea they do not think, 'I am the river Ganges,' or 'I am the river Kshipra.' They know, 'I am the sea.'

"In the same way, dear Shvetaketu, even though all creatures emerge from the ocean of consciousness, they do not know that. Whatever they are—whether tiger, lion, or wolf—in the end they return to the ocean of consciousness.

"That subtle essence of the whole world, the Self of all that is, the ocean of pure consciousness—that is truth. That is the Self, which unifies. Of that you are created. That thou art, Shvetaketu."

"Please, dear Father, teach me still more," Shvetaketu said.

"As you wish, my son," said his father. "Bring me a fruit from the banyan tree."

Shvetaketu went outside and picked a fruit from the long branches of the banyan tree. "Here it is, Father," said Shvetaketu.

"Break it open," said his father. "Tell me, what do you see inside?"

"I see many seeds."

"Break one seed open," said his father. "Tell me what you see."

"I see nothing at all," said Shvetaketu.

"My son, that 'nothing' is the subtle essence of all living things, which appears as nothing because you cannot perceive it. But from that nothing this great and ancient tree has grown.

"That infinite source of the whole universe, the Self of all that is, the ocean of pure consciousness—that is truth. That is the unmanifest Self. Of that you are created. That thou art, Shvetaketu."

"Please, honored Sir, teach me more," said Shvetaketu.

"As you wish, my dear son," said his father. "Fill this glass with water and add some salt. Then bring it to me in the morning."

Shvetaketu did this. The next morning his father said, "Bring me the salt you poured into the glass."

Shvetaketu returned with the glass of water and said, "The salt has disappeared, Father."

"Please take a sip from the top of the glass," his father said. "How does it taste?"

"Salty."

"Now pour out some and take a sip from the middle," said his father. "How does it taste?"

"It tastes salty."

"Now pour out some and take a sip from the bottom. Tell me, how does it taste?"

"Salty," said Shvetaketu.

"Even though you couldn't see it, the salt was found in every drop of water. In the same way, pure consciousness is found in all beings. That subtle essence of the whole world, the Self of all that is, the ocean of pure consciousness—that is truth. That is the all-pervading Self. Of that you are created. That thou art, Shvetaketu."

"Please, honored Sir, teach me more."

"As you wish, my dear son," said his father. "Think of a man left blindfolded in a desert. He wanders around, not knowing where to go. But if someone removes the blindfold and points out the right direction, he finds his way until finally he reaches home. In the same way, if a teacher points the way to Self-knowledge, then you enjoy the path to enlightenment—from the very first step you grow in intelligence, happiness, and success in life.

"That subtle essence of the whole world, the Self of all that is, the ocean of pure consciousness—that is truth. That is the Self, which removes the darkness of ignorance. Of that you are created. That thou art, Shvetaketu.

"When you have known this subtle essence of life, then you

have seen the unseen and known the unknown. You have known that by knowing which everything else becomes known."

And then Shvetaketu understood the true teaching of the Veda. Even when he later became a famous teacher in the court of King Janaka, Shvetaketu always remained humble, once he had realized the Self, the ocean of pure consciousness.

Chhandogya Upanishad, 6.1-18

"There is a light which shines beyond the world,
beyond everything, beyond all, beyond the highest heaven.
This is the light which shines within your heart."
Chhandogya Upanishad, 3.13.7

How Your Consciousness Affects Your Child

As your mental, physical, and emotional well-being develop through the Maharishi Transcendental Meditation^{SM} technique, the first beneficiary will be your child. After all, your child's health, starting from the moment the sperm and ovum unite, is directly influenced by your and your husband's consciousness. When you are the healthiest, happiest, and most loving, you can give the child the most nourishment—even at the time of conception.

And once you are pregnant, your mental and physical well-being will continue to affect your baby. In medical terms, the relationship between mother and baby is called "entrainment." You could think of it as a kind of tuning—the baby becomes attuned to the mother in the womb.

Entrainment is the tendency of natural cycles to come into coordination with each other. For example, if you put ten pendulums in a room, no matter how disparate the rhythms are when they start, they will eventually synchronize. In other words, they will entrain. Many people feel that the concept of bonding represents the biological rhythms of the baby seeking to entrain with those of the mother. It is known, for example, that a baby's breathing entrains with the mother's.

In other words, if you are happy and contented, your baby will be happy and contented even in the womb. This effect has been studied in newborns by measuring "Quiet Alert" periods. These are times when the baby is awake, alert, bright-eyed, and peaceful. (Infants are considered to be most receptive to learning while in this alert, contented state.) According to one research project, mothers who were practicing the Transcendental Meditation technique during their pregnancy gave birth to babies who exhibited this quiet alertness more than twice as much as comparable babies born to nonmeditating mothers. So the experience of feel-

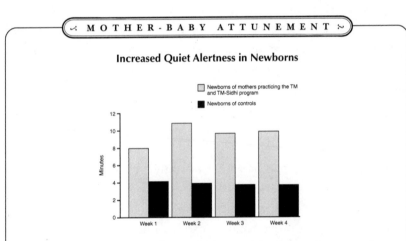

⌁ M O T H E R - B A B Y   A T T U N E M E N T ⌁

Increased Quiet Alertness in Newborns

An experimental group of 15 babies aged 1 month or younger, born to mothers practicing the Transcendental Meditation and TM-Sidhi programs, and a control group of babies born to non-meditating mothers, were matched according to gender, birth-order, diet, mother's lifestyle, and 21 other variables which have been related to the occurrence of Quiet Alert periods. These periods lasted more than twice as long in newborns in the experimental group (average duration 8.8 minutes), compared with the control group (average duration 3.3 minutes).

Reference: M.J. Doan, "Transcendental Meditation Program as a Prenatal Factor in the Quiet Alert State in Normal Newborns," paper presented at the Annual Meeting of the National Association of Young Children (November 1988).

ing more settled, combined with the exceptionally deep rest provided by the Transcendental Meditation technique, appears to aid the natural and profound relationship that develops between mother and baby. This may be the reason so many mothers find that practicing the Transcendental Meditation technique really helps to deepen the bond between themselves and their babies.*

And once your baby is born, you will need to draw on all your inner reserves to care for your new child. Everyone has heard of mother's intuition, how a mother naturally knows what her baby needs. And surely if you are feeling rested, alert, and free of stress, you can more easily provide that loving, tender care that so deeply nourishes your child.

Nancy started the Transcendental Meditation technique before conceiving her second child. *"What helped me the most was just resting as much as possible and practicing the Transcendental Meditation technique. The biggest problem for me in my first pregnancy was that I would get so anxious and think of all the million things I had to do, and I'd be running around much more than I should. I was much calmer with the second child, and my daughter was much more relaxed than my first child after birth."*

As your family grows, it's so important for you to be contented and flowing in love, because the mother is the center of the whole family. If you are healthy, blissful, and free of fatigue, you can give so much more to all those who depend on you. My patients who practice the Transcendental Meditation technique are so delighted with the extra energy and happiness they gain that they continue meditating twice a day as their children grow older.

"When they nap I meditate," says JoAnne, a busy mother of three.

---

* For those mothers who are already practicing the Transcendental Meditation technique, be sure to have your meditation checked by a qualified teacher of the Transcendental Meditation program, as there are special guidelines for pregnancy. If you would like to learn the Transcendental Meditation technique, see Appendix C for help in finding a teacher near your home.

"And my oldest child baby-sits while I'm meditating. The extra rest helped tremendously with postpartum recovery, and I've continued meditating twice a day all these years. I think it's nice to incorporate into the children's attitude that mother needs time to herself for her own growth. I tell them I can be a much sweeter person if I have time to myself to meditate, and they like me to do it.

"I also tell my children that I want to do this for my own peace and for the peace of the world. I think it's nice for them to be reminded of that, that we're creating peace in our hearts, peace in our family and peace in the world while we're meditating. It's a major contribution we can all make, and considering the condition of the world, it's important for me to do that. I let them know that I have a purpose in what I'm doing, and I want them to grow up with that in their awareness."

Summary

By enlivening consciousness and reducing stress, the Transcendental Meditation technique can help you nourish your baby during conception, pregnancy, postpartum, and throughout life.

"He whose mind-body principles are in balance, whose appetite is good, whose tissues are functioning normally, whose waste products are in balance, and whose body, mind, and senses remain full of bliss, is called a healthy person."   — *Shushruta Samhita*[11]

"When in a normal state, the mind-body principles are responsible for the maintenance of the health of the individual. So a wise man should try to keep them in their normal state."   — *Charaka Samhita*[12]

"Whichever parts of a pregnant woman get afflicted by the imbalance of the mind-body principles, the same parts of the fetus also get afflicted."
                          — *Sushruta Samhita*[13]

CHAPTER THREE

Nurturing the True Nature of Your Baby

Having a baby makes you feel so much a part of nature. Many women feel that the miracle of giving birth reveals their own essential nature—the part of themselves that can create new life.

To me, one of the most intriguing principles of the Maharishi Vedic Approach to Health is that human nature is a reflection of nature itself. The same remarkable intelligence that permeates and maintains order throughout the entire universe is found at the basis of human physiology. That same remarkable intelligence comes into play every time we create new life. Those same laws of nature permeate and maintain order in the growing embryo just as they do for the universe as a whole.

I like to think of every baby as a "cosmic baby," because every baby truly reflects the vast intelligence and creativity contained in a star, in a galaxy, in the entire cosmos. The 100 billion neurons active in a newborn's brain are as miraculous as the 100 billion stars of the milky way. As every newborn grows to childhood and adulthood, he or she has the ability to develop his or her infinite potential and to reflect the miraculous creative forces of our universe.

The Cosmic Baby

When a child is born, he owns in his genes the potential to be cosmic, to enjoy a life of vast intelligence, perfection and orderliness.

In Chapter One you learned about the discovery of Tony Nader, M.D., Ph.D., which revealed that the human physiology has inherent in it the full range of natural law. The same laws of nature that give form to the universe, that are expressed in the Veda and Vedic Literature, also give form to the human mind and body. The human body is the material expression of natural law, built and modelled on the basis of the same laws of nature that structure the whole universe and which are expressed in verbal form in Veda and the Vedic Literature. As such, the human body forms an exact replica of the patterns of intelligence that are expressed in the forty aspects of the Veda and Vedic Literature. In fact, says Maharishi Mahesh Yogi, the human physiology *is* Veda, the expression of Total Knowledge. It has the total potential of natural law available to it. No other living being on earth has this capability to enliven the laws of nature inherent in the brain physiology and to enjoy higher states of consciousness.

The brain of a human baby develops in a series of perfectly ordered steps. Think of this: Around the third week of embryonic development, a thin layer of cells folds into a fluid-filled hollow space called the neural tube. The cells in the neural tube multiply faster than we can even conceive of—at a rate of 250,000 cells per minute. Next these cells must move to various positions in the developing brain and begin forging the connections that will eventually link different parts of the brain together. Think of the intelligence necessary to create this transformation from a hollow tube to the human brain of an Einstein or Mozart.

Yet it's clear that some people use more of their full potential than others. Some people spontaneously act in accord with the laws of nature, and live their lives of intelligence, happiness, and success. Others use less of their full potential and suffer from ill health, unclear thinking, and lack of success. If every baby is cosmic, what causes some to become Mozarts or Einsteins while others struggle to survive? Is the main influence *nature* or *nurture*?

Research on the growth and development of infants shows that the human brain develops in an exquisite dance between the two. Neuronal connections are highly influenced by the stimuli that the baby is exposed to. Depending on the stimuli, certain neural connections get established in the brain early in life and become part of what makes up the individual's intelligence and personality. If these connections are not forged correctly, or if they are never corrected, the individual cannot make use of his or her full potential.

Consider this: Just ten or twelve weeks after conception, any slight stimulus to the fetus causes nerve cells in the developing brain to transmit waves of neural activity. This highly coordinated barrage of firing neurons actually changes the shape of the emerging brain, forming permanent neural patterns. The neural pathways forged in the womb allow the newborn baby to recognize its mother's voice and respond to her loving touch.

The environment continues to shape the brain after birth. In the critical first few years, the human brain begins producing trillions of extra connections between neurons—far more than it can possibly use. Depending on the sensory and emotional stimuli the child receives, the brain starts a process of eliminating the connections that are seldom or never used. The unused synapses are eventually weeded out, creating a unique pattern of emotions and thoughts in the brain. Thus the environmental stimuli do in fact determine which synapses are formed and which become dormant.

This means that any kind of sensory or emotional experience leaves a trail in the brain. If the stimulus is repeated over and over, the neurons get transformed permanently. At the same time, if there is a lack of proper stimulation at a particular point in the baby's development, the necessary connections do not get made, and the full development of the child could be delayed or hampered.

From the perspective of Maharishi Vedic Medicine, every baby has the potential to be cosmic, but this potential has to be developed by exposing the baby to the right stimuli. All of the programs of Maharishi Vedic Medicine aim to unfold the full potential of the human physiology, to provide the proper and timely sequence of exposure to the most appropriate stimuli for the full development of human life.

One program, in particular, involves listening to and reading the sounds of the Veda and the Vedic Literature to enliven the different aspects of the physiology. Because the brain and body are made of the same impulses of natural law that form the Veda and Vedic Literature, their sounds enliven their full expression in the individual. So the Maharishi Vedic Approach to Health looks beyond mere physical health, and provides programs that make it completely possible to develop higher states of consciousness, to learn to speak and act in accord with natural law, and to never make mistakes. Perfect health means living cosmic life: a life free of problems and suffering, a life as perfect as the cosmos itself. This is the aim of all of the programs of Maharishi Vedic Medicine, to raise the life of every individual to the divine.

The Building Blocks found in Nature and in Your Body

At a more concrete level, the Maharishi Vedic Approach to Health identifies the essential building blocks that make up the world (earth, water, fire, air and space)—and these same building blocks form the human body. There is a very intimate connection between individual and nature.

Maharishi Vedic Medicine locates three basic mind-body principles found in nature and the human body. These main organizing principles of nature, called *doshas*, are *Vata, Pitta*, and *Kapha*. Each of these three doshas has specific qualities:

- **Vata** is composed of air and space and is moving, quick, light, cold, rough, and dry.

- **Pitta** is composed of fire and water and is hot, sharp, light, acidic, and slightly oily.
- **Kapha** is composed of earth and water and is heavy, slow, steady, solid, cold, sweet, sticky, oily, and dull.

How are these found in nature? One example that is easy to identify is the seasons. Vata is the predominant principle operating in the cold, dry, windy winter. Pitta is most expressed during the hot, humid summer. And Kapha is found in the cool, wet spring.

In your body, these same doshas are found governing different functions. For example, the quickly moving Vata governs all movement, from the blinking of your eye to the circulation of your blood, to the movement of your baby down the birth canal. The fiery Pitta governs digestion and metabolism. And the heavy, wet Kapha governs the structure, bones, and fluids.

These three doshas originate at the deepest, most silent level of the mind and the most refined level of the body. While every person has all three doshas (you can see that all three are essential just to keep your body running at all), we each have a natural balance of Vata, Pitta, and Kapha in different proportions. Some people may have more Pitta, for instance, and others more Vata. If you walk quickly, talk quickly, and think quickly, those would be indications of more of the quick-moving Vata. If you have a sharp intellect and a strong digestion, these are indications of the fiery Pitta in your body. Or maybe you are slow-moving and have a muscular build, which would indicate the presence of the slow, heavy Kapha.

The three doshas do not remain fixed but are constantly in fluctuation. They can also become imbalanced. Unsuitable foods, stressful lifestyles, and even extreme weather can cause imbalance in the doshas. If these imbalances develop and are not corrected, they can lead to ill-health and disease.

At Maharishi Ayur-Veda Health Centers and Maharishi Vedic

Medical Centers, physicians analyze a person's natural state of balance in the functioning of Vata, Pitta, and Kapha and identify specific imbalances if they exist.

This assessment is very important, because differences in the natural balance and imbalance of the doshas create different health needs. A person with more Vata, for instance, will feel healthier eating different foods than a person who has more Kapha. Based on this assessment of the doshas, each person receives an individualized diet, exercise program, daily routine, herbal remedies, and other natural recommendation to keep the body in harmony with nature. There is never a blanket prescription. Every person is unique, and is treated for her specific health needs.

How does a physician or other health practitioner trained in Maharishi Vedic Medicine determine whether any imbalances have arisen that require specific approaches and treatments? One of the primary diagnostic tools is called pulse diagnosis, which was mentioned in Chapter One. The properly trained physician/ practitioner also examines dozens of characteristics, including body size and shape; muscular development and fat distribution; skin color and texture; hair, nails, and facial features; the walking speed; and the quality of voice and gestures. The kind of weather you like best, sleep patterns, food choices, your memory, and your reaction to stressful situations—all these contribute to a total picture of your mental, physical, and emotional health.

What is the Nature of Vata, Pitta, and Kapha?

You may feel that one of the three doshas—Vata, Pitta, or Kapha—describes you perfectly, in which case that particular dosha is probably predominating in your mind-body system. Or you may recognize a combination of elements from two or even all three. All three interact to create your unique nature. See if you can find yourself in any of these three descriptions.

VATA

WHEN IN BALANCE	WHEN OUT OF BALANCE
Vibrant, lively	Restless, unsettled
Clear and alert mind	Light, interrupted sleep
Flexible, resilient	Easily fatigued
Imaginative, sensitive	Constipated
Cheerful, optimistic	Anxious, worried
Regular habits	Underweight

WHAT CAUSES AN IMBALANCE IN VATA	HOW TO KEEP VATA IN BALANCE
Irregular routine	Maintain a regular routine.
Staying up late	Go to bed early.
Cold, dry weather	Eat three warm meals a day.
Excessive mental work	Drink plenty of warm liquids; avoid
Traveling	stimulants.
Accident or injury	Dress warmly; take warm baths.
	Choose calm, quiet
	environments.

PITTA

WHEN IN BALANCE	WHEN OUT OF BALANCE
Warm, loving, contented	Skin rashes, disease
Enjoys meeting challenges	Prematurely gray or thinning hair
Strong digestion	Irritable, angry, and impatient
Efficient in activity	Demanding, critical, excessively
Articulate and precise in speech	perfectionist
Sharp intellect	Heartburn, ulcers, digestive problems
	Finds hot weather unbearable

WHAT CAUSES AN IMBALANCE IN PITTA:	HOW TO KEEP PITTA IN BALANCE:
Excessive heat or exposure to the sun	Practice moderation in all things.
Time pressure, stressful deadlines	Take time for leisure; enjoy beauty in
Excessive activity, overwork	the environment.
Skipping meals	Avoid being outside or exercising
Alcohol, smoking	during the hottest part of the day.
Eating excessive amounts of sour,	Eat your largest meal at noontime.
salty, and pungent (spicy) foods	Avoid stimulants.

KAPHA

WHEN IN BALANCE	WHEN OUT OF BALANCE
Strong, vital energy	Complacent, dull, lethargic
Affectionate, generous, kind, forgiving	Oily skin, allergies, congestion
Solid, powerful build	Slow digestion, tendency to gain
Natural resistance to disease	weight
Good memory	Possessive, emotionally attached
Full of dignity and courage	Intolerant of the cold and damp
	Inability to accept change

WHAT CAUSES AN IMBALANCE IN KAPHA	HOW TO KEEP KAPHA IN BALANCE
Oversleeping	Don't oversleep.
Overeating	Don't overeat.
Eating too many heavy, sweet or oily foods	Include more hot spices in your food.
Insufficient exercise	Enjoy variety in life.
Not enough variety in life	Exercise regularly and vigorously.
Cold, wet weather	Stay warm; avoid the cold and damp.

Consulting a Physician Trained in Maharishi Vedic Medicine for Conception, Pregnancy, or Postpartum

If you consult a physician/practitioner trained in Maharishi Vedic Medicine for conception, pregnancy, or postpartum, he or she will advise you to seek the advice of an obstetrician for primary care. At the same time, you will receive recommendations to complement the advice of your medical doctor. The two systems of health care go hand-in-hand, each supporting the other. (Throughout this book, the term "physician/practitioner" will be used in reference to professionals who are trained in Maharishi Vedic Medicine. Terms such as family doctor, obstetrician, or pediatrician refer to fully trained medical doctors, but not necessarily trained in Maharishi Vedic Medicine.)

For a couple wanting to conceive, I would first determine any imbalances they each may have, and then give them the tools they need to bring their bodies back into balance. This would include specific recommendations concerning diet, exercise, behavior, and daily routine. Although these would be individually prescribed, there are certain recommendations that apply particularly to pregnancy. This is because conception, pregnancy, and postpartum are all governed by a subdivision of Vata dosha, called *Apana Vata.*

Childbirth itself is also governed by Apana Vata. However, for legal reasons, in the U.S. physicians trained in Maharishi Vedic Medicine do not offer Vedic recommendations for childbirth. In India, of course, physicians/practitioners trained in Maharishi Vedic Medicine offer primary care for conception, pregnancy, childbirth, and the postpartum period. Pulse diagnosis and herbal formulas are used to help the mother strengthen her body, correct imbalances, and nourish the baby at all stages of development. Pulse diagnosis is even used to ascertain the gender of the baby before birth.

Whether practicing in India or the U.S., I would continue to see the wife throughout her pregnancy and postpartum period, because there are many recommendations—including an extensive program for postpartum—that could help her feel more comfortable and happy during this critical time of life.

How Apana Vata Maintains Optimal Conditions of the Uterus and Surrounding Organs for Healthy Pregnancy

To understand the birthing process from the point of view of Maharishi Vedic Medicine, you need to grasp the principle of Apana Vata. Apana Vata is one of five subdivisions of Vata dosha. Each dosha (Vata, Pitta, and Kapha) has five such "subdoshas," and each governs a different area of the body.

Since Vata controls movement, each of its five subdoshas directs a different type of movement originating in different areas of the body. *Prana Vata* is located in the brain, head, and chest; *Udana Vata* in the throat and lungs; *Samana Vata* in the stomach and intestines; *Apana Vata* in the colon and lower abdomen; and *Vyana Vata* is located throughout the body through the nervous system, skin, and circulatory system.

Apana Vata governs the downward-moving functions of the body, such as elimination, menstruation, and the movement of the baby down the birth canal during the birthing process. Virtually all functions of the uterus during menstruation, pregnancy, and delivery are controlled by Apana Vata. So is the growth and differentiation of different organs of the fetus.

That's why it's important to keep Apana Vata in balance. If it becomes either too strong or too weak it might cause problems in pregnancy. For example, if Apana Vata is not functioning normally, it can cause the position of the fetus to shift, leading to problems in delivery. It can also cause infertility.

For this reason, your physician/practitioner will take special care to help you keep Apana Vata in a state of equilibrium throughout conception, pregnancy, and postpartum. Most of the recommendations for foods to eat, exercise, daily routine, and special treatments such as oil massage aim to balance this important area. Once you understand the role of Vata and especially Apana Vata, it's easier to understand why you might experience certain physical, emotional, and mental symptoms and how you can keep this important mind-body principle healthy.

Anxiety during pregnancy, for instance, can be caused by too much Vata, and can be alleviated by eating foods that balance Vata and by resting more. And the tremendous fatigue, insomnia, and depression often associated with the postpartum period are also symptoms of Vata imbalance, brought on by the extreme exertion of giving birth. The Vedic texts prescribe simple, natural recommendations (see Chapter Nine) to alleviate fatigue and bring your system quickly back to normal.

Ronda, a mother of three, says, *"You feel very tired after going through pregnancy and childbirth—it's quite a huge strain on the body.*

What I found during the first week after giving birth was that I was so exhausted, so wired that I couldn't sleep. But after receiving a Vedic oil massage, the fatigue was gone. To have that extreme, agitated tiredness disappear was the most amazing thing to me. Once I relaxed with the massage, I was able to catch up quickly on the missed sleep."

Summary

When you consult a physician/practitioner trained in Maharishi Vedic Medicine, he or she will prescribe individual recommendations based on your particular constitution and imbalances. If you are seeking advice for conception, pregnancy, or postpartum care, you will receive additional recommendations specifically designed to maintain mental, physical, and emotional balance at this special time of your life.

"When a man with unimpaired sperm and a woman
with an unafflicted genital tract, ovum, and uterus
conceive, the soul along with the mind descends into
the zygote [fertilized egg] lodged inside the uterus.
This results in the formation of the embryo. It grows
unafflicted, being nourished by wholesome foods and
being managed with proper daily routine. Thereafter
the fetus is formed . . . endowed with the excellence of
strength, complexion, mental faculties, and
compactness for delivery in time [in the ninth or tenth
month]."   — *Charaka Samhita*[14]

CHAPTER FOUR

Healthy Conception for a Healthy Baby

The conception of your child is a blessing and a source of great joy. No doubt the news that you are expecting will arouse tender feelings in all those close to you. Conception is an expression of great love between you and your husband and, love is the driving force for nourishing your child through his or her entire life.

It's ideal to start planning your conception several months ahead of time by consulting a physician/practitioner trained in Maharishi Vedic Medicine. Both you and your husband want to take steps to optimize health, to produce healthier ovum and sperm and thus a healthier baby. Although this chapter describes ways to improve your health before you conceive, it also contains important information even if you are already expecting.

Influences on Conception

According to *Charaka Samhita*, which you will remember from Chapter One is a major text used by Maharishi Vedic Medicine, several factors contribute to healthy conception:

- healthy ovum and sperm
- nutritional fluids (mother's diet)
- the health of the womb
- timing (i.e., the mother's age and the time in her cycle that conception occurs)

All of these factors can be improved through proper health care, and thus you have an opportunity to take responsibility for the welfare of your children even before conception. Of course, you can see that most of these influences are associated with the mother. What you eat, drink, smell, feel, and think from the weeks before conception until the baby is delivered will influence your baby.

Charaka Samhita gives detailed descriptions of characteristics of healthy ovum and sperm, and how they can be affected by hereditary factors, lifestyle changes, dietary habits and disease. It also mentions that the fetus is composed of elements relating one-fourth to the father, one-fourth to the mother, one-fourth to the mother's food intake, and one-fourth to the soul or consciousness of the child. Let's look at these influences one by one.

Healthy Ovum and Sperm: The health of the parents, heredity, diet, and mental factors all play an important role in the formation of healthy ovum and sperm for conception. The Vedic texts give detailed descriptions of characteristics of healthy ovum and sperm, and how they can be affected by these factors.

According to the Maharishi Vedic Approach to Health, healthy sperm and ovum are produced as a result of all the other tissues in the body being properly formed. Starting with the *rasa*, or nutritive fluid, the different body tissues (plasma, blood, muscle, fat, bone, bone marrow, reproductive tissue) get formed in successive stages. If at any one point in the chain a tissue, or *dhatu*, does not get formed properly, it affects all the following tissues. Each tissue builds on the ones preceding it.

The reproductive tissue, called *shukra*, is the seventh and final tissue to be formed in this sequence, the culmination of a chain of transformations which must proceed properly. This is why Maharishi Vedic Medicine places such importance on balancing the whole body to create healthy ovum and sperm, and thus a healthy child.

The Vedic texts also point out that some of the child's organs

How the Dhatus Develop Sequentially to Form Shukra Tissue

rasa ➤ rakta ➤ mamsa ➤ meda ➤ ashti ➤ majja ➤ shukra

DHATUS	CORRESPONDING TISSUES
Rasa	nutritive fluids, chyle
Rakta	blood
Mamsa	muscle
Meda	fat
Asthi	bone
Majja	bone marrow and the nervous system
Shukra	reproductive tissue

are derived from the ovum, and others from the sperm. The skin, for instance, comes from the maternal side while the bones come from the paternal side. In addition, the child has its own consciousness or soul, which combines with the sperm and ovum. Without the soul, the sperm and ovum alone cannot create a child.

Health of the Womb: If a woman wants to conceive and comes to me for a consultation, I look at her overall health and then at her menstrual cycle. The Vedic texts give a lot of attention to the diet and regimen of women during menstruation, because if a woman takes care of herself during menstruation, she can help maintain a healthier ovum and can nourish the fetus better once conception takes place. It can't be emphasized enough how important the overall health of the mother, ovum, and womb is to the unborn child's health—physical, mental, and emotional.

During menstruation, it is important that a woman take adequate rest, eat foods that are light and easily digestible, and refrain from vigorous activity. The Vedic texts give detailed recommendations, and these are available from physicians trained in Maharishi Vedic Medicine. Sexual relations are not recommended at that time, because conception during this period may not result in a healthy fetus.

It's also important to correct any serious imbalances, as these could affect the ovum. Imbalances can be corrected through various modalities of Maharishi Vedic Medicine, such as proper diet, lifestyle, herbal preparations, and purification treatments.

Nutritive Fluid: The foods you eat are directly transformed into the rasa or nutritive fluid that nourishes your baby in the womb. They also affect the quality of reproductive tissue, the sperm and ovum. That's why it's so important for both you and your husband to eat a healthy diet to produce the healthiest baby. Because food plays such an important role in conception and pregnancy, Chapter Six is devoted to dietary recommendations for conception as well as for pregnancy.

Timing of Conception: The Vedic texts describe the mother's optimum age to be from twenty-five to thirty years. This is partly because at this age the mother's bones are still soft, and the cartilage and ligaments are more flexible, making the delivery easier. Also, younger parents still have youthful energy and strength by the time their child reaches the energetic teen years!

Today, of course, women are delivering healthy children well into their forties. Probably the best indicator for an older woman to use is whether her menstrual cycle is regular and healthy.

Timing also refers to planning the conception and birth of a child during the times when planetary influences are more auspicious. Maharishi Vedic Astrology recommendations help the couple enjoy the support of nature by planning the conception and birth during the times when there will be fewer obstacles. When you choose an auspicious time for conception, pregnancy and birth can be smoother, creating more harmony and happiness in the parents, which will be reflected in the life of the baby. If there has been a history of infertility or miscarriages, it can help to have a Maharishi Vedic Astrology consultation, to help determine a future time when it may be easier to conceive.

The optimum time to conceive is four to twelve days after the menstrual flow begins (which is generally the time of optimum fertility). In addition, the Vedic texts even describe how to use timing to plan the gender of your child—conceiving on certain days for a male child and other days for a female child.

Preparing for Conception

Now that you have a basic background in some of the factors that contribute to healthy conception, let's look at the kinds of recommendations that a physician/practitioner trained in Maharishi Vedic Medicine might give a couple planning to conceive.

Identify Individual Health Needs: The first thing the physician/practitioner would do is determine the couple's individual health needs. The doctor would use pulse diagnosis to identify the state of balance or imbalance for both husband and wife—paying special attention to keeping the woman's Apana Vata in equilibrium. If there were any detectable imbalances, the physician would prescribe specific recommendations for diet, daily routine, herbal supplements and other natural approaches to correct them and help maintain the balanced functioning of both spouses' mind-body systems.

Practice the **Transcendental Meditation** *Program:* This would be the most important recommendation to enliven the inner intelligence of the body and to help both husband and wife reduce mental, emotional, and physical stress. Even more importantly, this simple technique helps develop the healthiest and happiest state of mind and emotions.

I notice that my patients who practice the Transcendental Meditation program naturally are drawn to more positive influences, and automatically find harmful substances to be distaste-

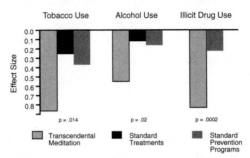

Reduced Drug and Alcohol Use

A statistical meta-analysis of 198 independent treatment outcomes found that the Transcendental Meditation program produced a significantly larger reduction in tobacco, alcohol, and non-prescribed drug use than substance abuse treatments and standard prevention programs. While effects of conventional programs typically fall off rapidly within 3 months, effects of the Transcendental Meditation program increase over time, with total abstinence from tobacco, alcohol, and non-prescribed drugs ranging from 51%-89% over a 18-22 month period.

References: 1. A. Royer, "The Role of the Transcendental Meditation Technique in Promoting Smoking Cessation: A Longitudinal Study," *Alcoholism Treatment Quarterly*, 11 (1/2) (1994).
2. E. Taub, S. Steiner, E. Weingarten, and K. Walton, "Effectiveness of Broad Spectrum Approaches to Relapse Prevention in Severe Alcoholism: A Long-Term, Randomized, Controlled Trial of Transcendental Meditation, EMG Biofeedback, and Electronic Neurotherapy," op. cit.
3. C.N. Alexander, M.A. Rainforth, and C.E. Robinson, "Treating and Preventing Alcohol, Nicotine, and Drug Abuse through the Transcendental Meditation Technique: A Review and Statistical Meta-analysis," in D.F. O'Connell and C.N. Alexander (editors), *Self Recovery—Treating Addictions Using Transcendental Meditation and Maharishi Ayur-Veda* (Binghamton, NY: Harrington Park Press, 1994); pp. 13-88.

Reduced Need for Hypertension Medication

In a report on cost-effective hypertension management, researchers compared the effectiveness of the Transcendental Meditation program and standard pharmaceutical treatments. Randomized studies indicated that the TM program reduced the predominant form of hypertension as effectively as five standard antihypertensive medications, and less expensively.

Reference: R.E. Herron, R.H. Schneider, J.V. Mandarino, C.N. Alexander, and K.G. Walton, "Cost-Effective Hypertension Management: Comparison of Drug Therapies With an Alternative Program," *The American Journal of Managed Care*, 2 (1996), pp. 427-437.

ful. In fact, research shows that smoking, drinking, and drug abuse naturally decrease as a person practices the TM® technique. Decreasing use of these harmful substances is better for your health at any time, but is especially important at the time of conception and pregnancy.

In addition, as people release stress and grow in health, they often find that they are able to use fewer drugs (both prescription and over-the-counter), especially for stress-related illnesses such as hypertension and asthma. This is especially helpful before and during pregnancy, as even medicines can have an effect on the sensitive fetus, and on conception itself. What better way to prepare for the birth of your baby than to learn to give your mind and body deep rest every day, and cleanse it of deep stresses and impurities?

Use Rejuvenation Therapies: Special purification and rejuvenation treatments called Maharishi Rejuvenation therapy are recommended for both husband and wife six weeks prior to conception. These include pleasant, natural, and gentle treatments such as warm oil massage, mild internal cleansing, and steam treatments. The idea is to cleanse the channels throughout the body, so toxins and impurities can be eliminated. Once these channels are clear, the body's natural intelligence can function without hindrance, revitalizing the entire system and improving energy, vitality, mental clarity, well-being, and resistance to disease. These treatments also help to strengthen and deeply nourish the tissues. It is said that when the husband and wife follow these purification procedures, they help create an unimpaired sperm, ovum, womb, and genital tract. Then there are no obstacles to conception, just as a spotlessly clean cloth can be dyed by a touch of color.[15]

Once you purify the body, then you can build it up and continue to nourish the tissues with healthy foods and other lifestyle recommendations. These rejuvenation treatments, available at many Maharishi Ayur-Veda Health Centers, have such a profound effect on the physiology that even some couples with a history of infertility problems are able to conceive after taking this program.

⊰ REVITALIZING THE PHYSIOLOGY ⊱

**Improvement in Cardiovascular Risk Factors
Through Panchakarma Purification Procedures**

Thirty-one subjects were evaluated before and after 3-5 days of Maharishi Rejuvenation therapy according to a variety of psychophysiological measures. Improvements included an acute reduction in cholesterol plus an improvement in its ratio to high-density cholesterol (HDL); reductions in pulse rate and diastolic blood pressure; and improvements in state anxiety measures. These results indicate a reduction in cardiovascular risk factors.

Reference: H.M. Sharma, S.I. Nidich, D. Sands, and D.E. Smith. "Improvement in Cardiovascular Risk Factors Through Panchakarma Purification Procedures," *The Journal of Research and Education in Indian Medicine*, 12 (4), (1993), pp. 3–13.

Eat a Nourishing Diet: A nourishing diet designed to build up shukra dhatu (the seventh, reproductive tissue) is the best. For mothers and fathers who are planning to conceive, Maharishi Vedic Medicine recommends certain foods: milk, raw sugar, *ghee* (clarified butter), almonds, cashews, dates, figs, raisins, fresh fruits and vegetables, cracked wheat cereal (bulgur wheat), whole grains, fresh fruit juices, and plenty of pure spring water. These foods have an inherent purity and will promote the health of the ovum and sperm. It is suggested that both parents include these wholesome foods in their diet for at least six weeks before conception.

You will also want to avoid processed foods, heavy foods such as red meat, chicken, fish, cheese, fatty foods, and sour foods. Garlic, onions, mushrooms, and fermented foods do not nourish the sperm and ovum and should be avoided as well.

Keep a Healthy Daily Routine: It's important to enter into pregnancy well rested. Besides meditating regularly and getting enough exercise and sufficient sleep at night, you may also want to add a daily self-massage to your morning routine. This has a rejuvenating yet relaxing effect that helps improve immunity and promotes healthier functioning of all the body's systems. (See Chapter Seven for a more in-depth description and explanation.)

Enjoy a Happy, Stable Relationship: Happy families spring from a happy relationship between husband and wife. The best thing you can do to make your child feel wanted and loved is to strengthen the bond between yourself and your husband.

Avoid Harmful Substances: It is now widely known that alcohol and cigarettes can be harmful to the fetus. If you are thinking of becoming pregnant, you'll want to stop using these right away. You'll want to be as healthy as possible when you conceive—and you'll want to protect your baby from harm during those vulnerable first months when all the major organs are being formed. Be sure to consult with your obstetrician about the safety of continuing any medications you may already be taking.

Charaka Samhita identifies most of these harmful influences, citing intoxicating beverages, meat, spicy foods, strenuous exercise, and influences that are unwholesome to the senses. These are unhealthy during pregnancy and can interfere with conception as well.

Additional Influences on Fertility

It is fascinating that the Maharishi Vedic Approach to Health is so complete that it even describes the kind of atmosphere that the husband and wife should generate at the time of conception. Recognizing the effect of the mind and emotions on the unborn child, the Vedic texts recommend a pure, clean, pleasant environment, with the husband and wife thinking uplifting thoughts, to attract a pure and high-minded soul. The surroundings should be pleasing

Harmful Substances to Avoid During Pregnancy

CIGARETTES

Aside from the obvious health risks to the mother, smoking deprives the baby of oxygen. Cigarette smoke has been linked with premature birth, low birth weight, miscarriage, birth defects, and other risks to the baby. Secondary smoke should also be avoided.

ALCOHOL

Doctors advise not drinking at all while you're pregnant, as alcohol can injure the developing child. According to Vedic texts, it has a very destructive effect on *ojas*, which is a health-giving substance that directly nourishes the reproductive tissue. (Ojas will be discussed in detail in Chapter Six). While milk is the substance most nourishing to ojas, alcohol is the most destructive.

MEDICATION AND DRUGS

Because even over-the-counter medications such as aspirin can have harmful effects on your baby, it's best to avoid medication of all kinds while you're pregnant. Always check with your doctor before taking any medication once you are pregnant. If you must take medication for an on-going health problem, consult your doctor before becoming pregnant to see if your dosage can be lessened. And of course nonprescription, recreational drugs (including alcohol and cigarettes) can have a damaging effect, and can even disrupt the DNA of the reproductive cells.

CERTAIN ANIMAL PRODUCTS

Cat and dog feces and raw meat can contain a parasite called toxoplasma, which can bring serious harm to the unborn child. Pregnant women should avoid emptying litter boxes and should wear gloves for gardening. Wash your hands after handling raw meat.

to all five senses, and both partners are advised to wear clean, pleasing apparel. Flowers, incense, and soothing music help to create a soft, receptive ambiance. There are also instructions for the best posture for healthy conception—and positions to avoid because they disturb Vata, Pitta, or Kapha.

It's especially important that the woman enjoy a pleasant, relaxed state of mind. Worry, fear, unhealthy diet, fasting, and grief are said to inhibit conception or produce unhealthy offspring. Most of all, a strong feeling of love and desire for each other is an important ingredient for healthy conception.

One of my patients, the mother of a 5-year-old son, came to me for a check-up after her second pregnancy ended in a miscarriage. Sandy, age 36, describes the result: *"Because of the miscarriage I really started taking better care of my body. I started following recommendations from the Maharishi Vedic Approach to Health, including a healthy diet, which was designed to bring my body back into balance. Each morning I treated myself to a special self-massage that helped my body eliminate impurities and build immunity. I made sure I got lots of rest. I knew that these were exactly what I needed to create a healthy baby. And not only did I conceive effortlessly, but my baby has been extremely healthy and happy."*

Summary

Planning for a baby is an exciting time of your life, when you want to be at the peak of health. By consulting a physician trained in Maharishi Vedic Medicine, you and your husband can improve your own physical and mental well-being—and in that way prepare for a healthy conception.

"The heart of the fetus, which is derived from the maternal source, is connected with the mother's heart through the channels carrying nutrient material. These channels, connecting the fetus and the mother, carry the desires of the one to the other. It is with this end in view that people do not want to ignore the desires of the fetus as reflected through the wishes of the pregnant mother. If such desires are ignored, it could harm the development of the fetus.

"The proper maintenance and protection of the pregnant mother is as good as the maintenance or protection of the fetus itself. So the wise attend upon a pregnant mother with special care to fulfill her favorite and useful needs." —*Charaka Samhita*[16]

CHAPTER FIVE

How Your Baby Will Develop During the Next Nine Months

After your baby is conceived, the embryo begins a series of dramatic changes over the course of nine months that will bring it from a single cell to a fully functioning human being. During the first month after conception alone, an embryo multiplies its size by 40 and its weight by 3000. It is one of the miracles of life that this amazing transformation takes place without you, the mother, having to consciously do anything. Nature takes care of every detail.

Today, researchers know which organs are developing during each week of the nine months. The Vedic texts *Charaka Samhita* and *Sushruta Samhita* also give detailed information about the different stages of the development of the fetus. It is very close to what modern researchers have discovered in recent years. Without high-tech imaging equipment such as ultrasound, the Vedic seers were able to cognize these processes of development from deep within their own consciousness.

According to the *Sushruta Samhita*, all the baby's organs develop simultaneously, but the rate of growth varies from organ to organ.

All parts and their subdivisions appear simultaneously.
Due to their minuteness, the sprout of a bamboo or
the fruit of the mango cannot be recognized [while in
the early stages of development].

It is like this—in due course of time, pollens, pulp, nut, and kernel are seen separately in a ripe mango; however, the same components are indistinguishable in the early stage because of their minuteness. Time alone makes the pollens and the other components obvious in due course. The same can be said about the sprout of the bamboo tree.

Similarly, in the early embryonic stage, even though all the parts and organs are present they are not perceptible because of their minuteness; the same components, however, become obvious in due course of time.[17]

This chapter describes the embryo's progress during each month of pregnancy—and compares the Vedic texts with modern obstetrics research.*

The First Month of Life

From **Charaka Samhita:** During the first month, the organs of the embryo remain unformed. After the union of the sperm and ovum at the time of conception, the embryo is said to have a jelly-like consistency. After about seven days, it looks like a bubble. The density increases slowly, and by the fifteenth day, the embryo becomes firm. The whole 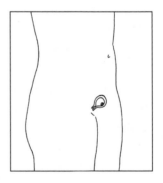 mass becomes hard by the end of the first month.[18]

From **Modern Obstetrics Research:** We know that the zygote, or single cell created by the fusion of sperm and ovum, begins to

---

*Please note that in modern obstetrics there are two ways to measure time of pregnancy: (1) The birth takes place approximately 280 days (forty weeks, which is equal to nine calendar months or ten lunar months) counting from the first day of your last menstrual cycle; or (2) the birth takes place approximately 266 days after conception. The Vedic texts use the first method, by counting ten lunar months, or forty weeks, measured from the first day of your last period.

divide almost immediately. It continues to divide as it travels down the fallopian tube and enters the womb. By the end of week three, the fertilized egg embeds itself in the thick lining of the womb. Once it is securely attached, sponge-like fingers from the embryo's outer cells sink into the lining, to link up with the mother's blood vessels. These later form the placenta.

The Second Month of Life

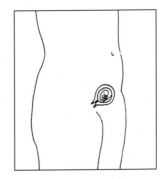

From **Charaka Samhita:** The shape of the embryo during this month gives an indication of the gender of the fetus. If the fetus is shaped like a knot and has a firm consistency, then the child is a male. If it is shaped like a muscle, the child is a female. If it is shaped like an egg, then the gender has not yet been differentiated.

From Modern Obstetrics Research: The embryo is floating in a fluid-filled sac by week five or six. The embryo has a simple brain, spine, and central nervous system. The digestive system, mouth, jaw, stomach, and chest are beginning to develop. The eyes and ears are just four shallow dimples on the head, and the limbs are four tiny buds.

The Third Month of Life

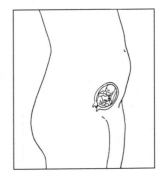

From **Charaka Samhita:** During the third month, all the sense organs and all the limbs emerge simultaneously. The fetal mass gives rise to five projections—two for the lower limbs, two for the upper limbs, and one for the head and neck. But the body parts are difficult to differentiate and identify. When the sense organs manifest and the latent mind activates, there is a throbbing sensation in the heart. This happens in the third month.

The heart is said to be the seat of consciousness. The heart of the fetus is connected with the placenta through the channels that carry nutrient material. The placenta in its turn is connected with the mother's heart through the arteries. Thus there is a direct link between the heart of the fetus and the heart of the mother.

And since the heart is the center for consciousness in the fetus, the feelings in the heart of the fetus are felt in the heart of the mother. The mother expresses the baby's feelings through her own feelings. She may crave different kinds of foods or want certain comforts or changes in her daily schedule. It is said that she is "two-hearted," which means that she now has to nourish and fulfill the desires of both her baby and herself.

It is very important to satisfy all of these longings, as otherwise the fetus will suffer physically or mentally. This is a key point in the Maharishi Vedic Approach to Health—because it points to the intimate connection between mother and baby. Caring for the mother is the same as caring for the unborn child. The mother should be given whatever she wants during this period, except those things that are harmful for the fetus.

From Modern Obstetrics Research: By the end of week six the heart—just a bump on the chest—starts beating. The heart starts to circulate blood throughout the body of the embryo by week seven. As for the sense organs, by the beginning of the third month a face can be discerned—nose, nostrils, mouth, and tongue can be identified. The inner parts of the ears (which control balance and hearing) start developing. By the end of the third month, all of the internal organs are formed, and most are functioning. The eyelids have developed, and are sealed over the eyes; the fetus has earlobes. The limbs are completely formed—

including fingers and toes, fingernails and toenails—but are proportionately smaller in comparison to the arms. The fetus can move his mouth muscles to frown, and to open and close his mouth. And he can curl his toes and make a fist. He responds to touch.

The Fourth Month of Life

From **Charaka Samhita:** During this month the fetus becomes more securely established, and the mother shows a pronounced increase in body weight. She may also feel a heaviness in her body, because the fetus becomes more compact, dense, and heavy. The different organs become more distinctly formed, and hair starts growing on the body.

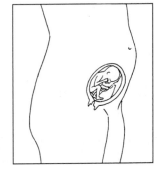

From Modern Obstetrics Research: The fetus grows rapidly during this month. He will grow from three and one-half inches to six inches; from one ounce to four ounces. Due to the rapid growth of the fetus during the second trimester (the fourth, fifth, and sixth months of pregnancy) you will gain more weight—up to 60 percent of your total pregnancy weight gain. You may feel healthier and more energetic during the second trimester and will probably begin to look pregnant and need looser clothing. Your appetite will probably increase as morning sickness subsides.

The fetus has a neck now and the head is still large in comparison to the body. The joints have formed in the arms and legs, and hard bones are beginning to develop. By now the heart is recirculating nearly twenty-five quarts of blood through the body per day. The heart muscle is strong. The fetal heartbeat is twice as rapid as yours—and you will probably be able to hear it through a stethoscope during this month. By week fourteen the placenta is developed enough to begin providing the fetus with nourishment.

The Fifth Month of Life

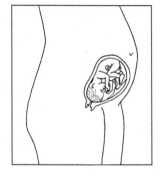

From **Charaka Samhita:** The weight of the fetus increases during this month due to an increase of flesh and blood. As the fetus increases in weight, the mother needs to be properly nourished or she will actually lose weight. After the fifth month, she gains weight more easily, although more slowly.

From Modern Obstetrics Research: The fetus grows to about eight inches and weighs about half a pound. The fetus has developed a fine, hairy covering known as *lanugo*. The sex organs are visible, although not always detectable by ultrasound. The fetus is probably very active, kicking and turning. You might experience this as a faint fluttering.

The Sixth Month of Life

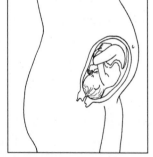

From **Charaka Samhita:** In comparison with the preceding months, the fetus grows in strength and vitality during this month. Consequently, the mother's strength and vitality can diminish during this period.

From Modern Obstetrics Research: Before the sixth month, the fetal head was curled forward and the abdomen bulged, causing the growing internal organs to be closely crowded. By the sixth month the fetus straightens out and becomes erect, exposing more of the skin surface of the body. From the sixth month, the skin starts changing from a red, wrinkled thin layer with little or no fatty deposits into a protective layer that can regulate its own temperature and protect itself against cold. Also, by the sixth month a grayish-white, cheesy coating (called *vernix*) covers the skin. This protects the fetus from abrasions when moving around and keeps the delicate skin from hardening in the mineralized amniotic fluid. By the end of the sixth month, sweat glands begin to form.

The fetus will grow to a length of about thirteen inches and weigh about one and one-fourth pounds during the sixth month. You'll feel the fetus moving around, kicking well-developed arm and leg muscles. At this stage, the unborn child can cough and hiccup. During this month you may gain as much as one pound per week.

The Seventh Month of Life

From **Charaka Samhita:** The fetus grows in all aspects. The pregnant woman begins to feel particularly tired and restless.

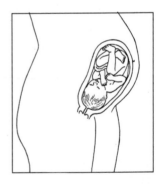

From Modern Obstetrics Research: The baby can now suck his thumb. At this time the unborn child has more taste buds than he will at the time of birth, and he can respond to sweet, sour, or acid tastes by making a face. Fat is starting to accumulate under the skin, making it less red and wrinkled. The brain develops dramatically during this month. Although his lungs are not fully mature, the baby could survive with special help if delivered during this month.

The Eighth Month of Life

From **Charaka Samhita:** A refined sub-stance called *ojas*, described in Vedic texts as the essence of the tissue elements of the body (see Chapter Six), transfers from the mother's body to the baby—and then flows back from the baby to the mother through the placenta. This fluctuation of ojas creates a wavering feeling of joy and sorrow in 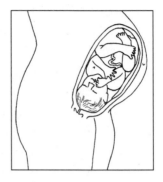 the mother. Because the ojas is unsteady during this month, there is more danger to the fetus.

That's why the Vedic texts recommend that the mother avoid traveling during the eighth month, to avoid any undue strain on the baby. The mother should be protected more at this time, sheltered from any shock, fear, or sadness. She should not be left alone, as she needs to be surrounded by love. A premature delivery at this time could prove life-threatening to the child.

From Modern Obstetrics Research: You will probably be feeling bulky and tired, so get all the rest you can. You may need to take rest breaks during the day. You may find that your emotions are swinging wildly, between longing for your baby to be born and feeling apprehensive about delivery and the responsibilities of motherhood.

The baby is now fully formed, and his head size is in proportion to the rest of his body. Your baby will grow to about sixteen inches in length and weigh around three and one-half pounds during this month. The weight gain of both mother and baby slows down.

The Ninth Month Onwards

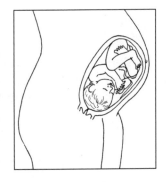

From **Charaka Samhita:** In most cases, delivery takes place in the tenth month. (Remember, we're counting every four weeks as one month.) Inside the womb, the fetus is said to lie with his face towards the back of the mother, having his head above and the limbs folded (until moving his head into the birth canal prior to delivery).[19]

From Modern Obstetrics Research: Your baby will have lost most of the lanugo hair and may still have traces of vernix. His skin will be plump and flesh-colored. His fingernails may be sharp and long enough to scratch himself. The intestines of the baby will accumulate *meconium,* a dark, sticky mass of cells and wastes. It will be passed in the baby's first bowel movements after birth. The fetus almost always shifts to a head-down position shortly before delivery. Just before full term, the rate of weight gain will slow and may even stop. By week forty, he will be about twenty inches long and weigh about seven and one-half pounds.

Summary

One of the most remarkable experiences is to feel your baby kicking and to hear his heartbeat. Knowing the baby's stages of development during the nine months following conception can help you understand what to expect and how to keep your pregnancy as smooth and comfortable as possible.

"The nutritive fluid (the digestive product of food) of the pregnant woman serves three purposes: nourishment of her own body, lactation, and growth of the fetus. Being supported by that food, the fetus who is dependent upon the mother keeps living inside.

"The fetus is free from thirst and hunger. It is dependent upon the mother for all its activities. . . . The heart of the mother floods the placenta with nourishment through the pulsating vessels. This nutritive fluid promotes strength and vitality of the fetus."   —*Charaka Samhita*[20]

CHAPTER SIX

Eating for Two

When you are pregnant, your diet becomes more important than ever before. After all, your baby's sole means of nourishment is through you. What you eat will directly affect your baby's health, so naturally you will want to eat only the purest, healthiest, and most wholesome foods. You will remember from Chapter Four that Maharishi Vedic Medicine emphasizes the mother's diet as one of the four important factors that determine the health of the child.

During pregnancy, the nutrient fluid formed by the digestion of food is used for three different purposes: to nourish the mother, to be deposited in the breast for use during breast-feeding, and to nourish the fetus. Pregnancy requires extra work from your body—and that's why you want to be sure that the food you eat is especially nourishing.

The good thing is that pregnancy is a time to really enjoy eating. You'll want to set aside extra time for preparing regular, hot meals. Skipping meals, eating on the run, fasting, and eating junk food can all reduce the nutrition your baby needs to grow normally.

You'll also want to eat soothing, easily digestible foods to nourish Vata dosha, the mind-body principle described in Chapter Three that is so important during pregnancy and childbirth.

When Vata is out of balance you can feel more anxious, worried, and weak, so Maharishi Vedic Medicine recommends foods that will calm, soothe, and strengthen you.

Fresh and Wholesome

To derive the most nutritional value from food, *eat lots of fresh vegetables and fruits, whole grains, and dairy products.* You will also want to avoid packaged foods, because these have so many additives that have no nutritional value. If at all possible, try to eat organic foods, to avoid exposing your baby to pesticides and chemicals during this important time of growth. "Eating organic" will also reduce your and your baby's exposure to new "high tech" foods that may have been irradiated or genetically engineered. Drinking lots of pure spring water will help flush any impurities out of your body.

A point often overlooked is that *food should be delicious.* You'll digest your food better if it's attractive and tasty, and has been prepared with love.

Maharishi Vedic Medicine also recommends that you eat balanced meals of *cooked* foods, since cooking the food makes it more soothing, nourishing, and easier to digest.

Food Cravings

The most important thing is to relax and enjoy eating. Everyone knows that pregnant women sometimes have unusual cravings, such as pickles and ice cream. As mentioned in Chapter Five, it is said in the Vedic texts that after the third month, the baby speaks to the mother through the mother's desire for food. When you really want to eat something, it's probably what your baby needs at that particular moment. If you deny yourself, you might actually deprive your baby of specific nutrients necessary for that particular stage of growth. So this is the time to eat what you want! It is said that if the expectant mother's longings are satisfied, then she will give birth to a healthy, strong, and virtuous child with a long life-span.[21]

You may also crave a larger amount of one or another food than is normal. For instance, for a few days you may want more green, leafy vegetables. This means that you or your baby needs those particular nutrients. But one precaution is that you still want to make sure your diet is genuinely balanced, as cravings can also be caused by an imbalanced diet.

What if you desire something that is not healthy? If the desire persists, you can eat just a small quantity of that food to satisfy your yearning, and eat it along with other healthy foods. One of the best ways to satisfy cravings is to eat a diet that has all six tastes.

A Balanced Diet with All Six Tastes

You are probably used to thinking of foods in terms of calories, and perhaps you think of a balanced diet as containing foods from all levels of the "food pyramid." Maharishi Vedic Medicine has a different way of classifying foods—according to six basic tastes. These are sweet, salty, sour, pungent, bitter, and astringent.

If you eat all of these six tastes, you will notice that your body will feel more nourished and satisfied. If you habitually ignore some of these tastes, you may develop intense cravings or insatiable hunger, and may feel unsatisfied at the end of a meal. Eating a balanced diet means including these tastes in every meal.

What are some examples of these tastes? You probably will recognize the sweet, salty, and sour tastes right away, since most Americans eat a lot of those tastes in the form of desserts (sweet), salty snacks (salty), and vinegar (sour). But you may be surprised to find that these tastes also appear in healthy food.

For example, sweet foods include milk, unsalted butter, ghee (clarified butter), rice, wheat, pasta, bread, and sweet fruits.

The sour taste is found in yogurt and other cultured dairy

products, and in lemons, grapefruits, and other sour fruits.

The salty taste is found, obviously, in mineral, sea, or table salt—but it also occurs naturally in many vegetables.

Pungent foods are hot and spicy. They include cayenne, chili peppers, black pepper, radishes, cumin, and ginger.

You may not be as familiar with the other two tastes, astringent and bitter. "Astringent" means "dry," so astringent foods include beans, lentils, dahl, pomegranates, persimmons, spinach, cabbage, broccoli, and cauliflower.

And bitter tastes include bitter greens such as endive, chicory, and parsley, as well as leafy greens such as kale, spinach, chard, and collard greens. Sprouts and bitter gourd also have bitter tastes.

Each of these foods has an effect on the body. For instance, sweet tastes are heavy and nourishing. Sour, salty, and pungent tastes stimulate digestion. Bitter and astringent tastes lighten and cool the body.

As already mentioned, all six tastes should be included in every meal, but the unique genius of Maharishi Vedic Medicine is that diet can be tailored to correct specific imbalances in your body. In other words, different types of people have different health needs, and they need to eat the specific foods that will make them feel healthiest. You'd still eat all six tastes, but you'd include more of the tastes that your particular mind-body system needs. In fact, you might find yourself naturally favoring those tastes.

A person who is lethargic or heavy, for instance, might feel stimulated by pungent-tasting foods. Someone with a more fiery nature would feel better eating more cooling foods, such as the astringent and bitter tastes. People who are very active and light, with thoughts spinning around in their heads, may need settling, sweeter foods to make them feel more stable. And particular imbalances you may have could require additional fine-tuning.

Your physician/practitioner trained in Maharishi Vedic Medicine will outline the foods that are best for you, after taking into account your nature and imbalances. For many pregnant women, the sweet, sour, and salty tastes are best. This is because these foods are most nourishing for both mother and baby, helping supply the extra calories and building nutrients to form new life.

Of course, you don't want to be compulsive about eating these recommended foods, but it's easy to include them in your diet.

Although eating sweet foods is best during pregnancy, this doesn't mean you should eat lots of refined sugar. Rather, it means favoring sweet foods such as milk, ghee, rice, and wheat. If

---

Recommended: Sweet, Sour, and Salty Foods for Pregnancy

In General: Eat more warm, cooked, unctuous (oily) food and warm drinks. Eat all six tastes, but reduce highly pungent, bitter, and astringent tastes. Favor sweet, salty, and sour tastes. Stay away from uncooked foods and cold foods and drinks, as these tend to extinguish the "digestive fire."

Dairy: Whole milk, butter, freshly made yogurt, fresh cheeses such as panir, ricotta, or cottage cheese.

Sweeteners: Honey, natural sugar (in moderation).

Oils: Olive oil, ghee (clarified butter).

Fruits: Sweet, fresh, ripe, room-temperature fruits such as papaya, coconut, peaches, mangoes, sweet pineapple, sweet oranges, sweet plums, sweet berries, and sweet apples. Raisins and dates are especially nourishing for the fetus.

Vegetables: Beets, carrots, zucchini, sweet potatoes or yams, peeled cucumbers, spinach, squash, peeled eggplant, asparagus.

Grains: Rice, pasta, whole-grain bread, millet, quinoa, and other whole grains.

Beans: Yellow split mung dahl (available in natural food stores or Indian grocery stores), tofu.

Spices: Fenugreek, fennel, saffron, cinnamon, cardamom, cumin, ginger, salt, clove, mustard seed, small amounts of black pepper.

Nuts: Blanched almonds are especially nourishing for the fetus.

---

you crave desserts, it's fine to eat them—in moderation. But keep in mind that these are empty calories and eating too many desserts could keep you from eating nutritional foods. Also, chocolate has caffeine and should be avoided.

What is Ideal Digestion?

The interesting thing about eating is that *what* you eat is only half the story. In the Maharishi Vedic Approach to Health, *how* you eat is considered even more important. This is because digesting the food, actually making use of the nutrients you take in, is really the goal of eating. And never is it more important that you make good use of your food than when you are nourishing your unborn baby.

Let's say you sit down to eat a sumptuous, nutritious, deliciously prepared banquet. Yet you can't derive nourishment from it if your digestion is weak. On the other hand, if your digestion is strong, you can still extract great value from the food even if it isn't the very best.

What are the signs of ideal digestion? One indication is how you feel after you eat. If your digestion is working well, you will feel light, happy, and satisfied after a meal. If it is weak, you may feel uncomfortable, have gas or pain, or feel dull. Another sign is your overall health, mental and physical.

There are two principal players in the drama of digestion. The digestive fire (called *agni* in the Vedic texts) is the force that transforms the food into the living cells of your body, and now that you are pregnant, into the living cells of your baby's body. From the moment your food is swallowed it goes through a series of transformations that allows it to nourish and build the seven body tissues (plasma, blood, muscle, fat, bone, bone marrow, and reproductive tissue).

This transforming fire, agni, is the bright hero of the drama of digestion. When it is burning brightly and steadily, like a well-tended fire in your fireplace, then digestion takes place normally. When it is diminished for any reason (by eating too much, eating foods that are too hard to digest, or by disruptions to the meal) then it is just as if you had put too many logs in your fireplace and smothered the flame.

When this happens, then the food is left in your stomach undigested, and waste products begin to accumulate in your digestive track. This undigested food (called *ama* in the Vedic texts) has the opposite qualities of the fiery agni. Cold and sticky, a toxic waste-product of digestion, it collects in the tissues and creates imbalances wherever it spreads. In short, it's the enemy to good health. These toxic impurities accumulate in the stomach, cells, and tissues, and are actually the seeds of future disease. That is why keeping digestion running smoothly is such an important part of Maharishi Vedic Medicine.

To Keep Your Digestion Running Smoothly

How do you keep your digestion healthy? Digestion is a natural process, and having a healthy digestion is a result of living in tune with natural law. If you listen to your body's signals, eat at the times of day when your digestive fire is naturally turned up high, chances are your digestion is already strong.

Unfortunately, most people today are living a lifestyle that is completely out of tune with nature. Many people eat lightly at noon, when digestion is actually at its peak, and eat their heavy meal right before bed, when the digestive fire is dimmest. In American cities, it's common to see busy people eating on the run, consuming fast food while driving in their cars or even while walking down the street. Busy moms sometimes jump up many times during a meal, never really settling down to digest the food.

Fortunately, Maharishi Vedic Medicine offers many practical suggestions for improving your digestion. *Charaka Samhita* gives the following advice:

One should take wholesome food at regular, timely
intervals. Further, one should eat warm, unctuous
food, in the proper quantity, after the previous meal is
digested. The food should be eaten in a favorable
place, should not be eaten too fast, too slowly, or with
excessive talking or laughing, but with the full
attention, presence of mind, and after due
consideration to the Self.[22]

This passage contains a lot of wisdom. If you eat your main
meal at noon, for instance, you'll digest the food more easily. This
is because there is a correlation between the agni in your body
(the digestive fire) and the agni in nature (the sun). The sun is
strongest at noon every day, when the sun is at its peak in the sky.
This is the time the digestive fire in your body is also at its peak.
By eating the main meal at noon, you take advantage of the full
strength of agni to digest the food. If you ignore this natural cycle
and eat the heaviest meal at night, it can result in undigested
food and accumulated ama. The same can be said about heavy
foods in general: It's better not to strain your agni by eating them
at night, including meat, cheese, or other cultured foods. Breakfast should be lighter than the noon meal, too, as your digestive
fire takes time to wake up in the morning.

Keep in mind that it takes most people at least three hours to
digest a large meal. You don't want to start eating again until the
previous meal is digested. Think what would happen if you
started to cook some beans, and after half an hour you added
some raw beans to the partially cooked ones. You'd end up with a
sticky, gluey mess before the new beans got cooked. In the same
way, eating before the last meal is digested can interrupt the digestive process and create ama.

Of course, when you are pregnant, you may be hungry more
often, and it's important to respond to your desires and cravings
since these are your baby's desires. You can aim to eat regular

meals, but if you feel hungry more often than that—be sure to follow your desires. Also, some women find that in the later months, their stomach capacity grows smaller as the baby grows bigger, so eating smaller, more frequent meals can work better.

Taking time to taste your food is more important than you might think. Digestive juices start flowing when you see attractive food, and when it reaches your taste buds the stomach starts preparing to digest. Savor all the six tastes, and your digestion will be stronger. It helps if you don't distract yourself by watching TV, listening to music, reading, or doing business over a meal. Keeping the conversation light and enjoyable can actually help your digestion.

It's really important to sit down when you eat, as standing can put a strain on digestion and disrupt it. If you're a busy mother with several young children, try to eat after the children are finished or set everything on the table first so you don't have to jump up so much. It also helps digestion get off to the right start if you remain sitting comfortably and quietly for a few minutes after the meal.

While you'll never want to fast, eat too little, or skip a meal while pregnant, you'll also want to avoid overeating. Overeating can cause uncomfortable gas or indigestion, which pregnant mothers often experience. Be sure to follow your obstetrician's advice for weight gain during pregnancy.

For a deeper understanding of the Vedic principles associated with diet, I recommend a sixteen-hour course on diet, digestion, and nutrition developed by Maharishi Vedic University. See Appendix C for details.

The Finest Product of Digestion

When digestion is running smoothly, and there is a minimum of ama, your body will create more of a subtle substance called *ojas* (introduced in Chapter Five). Ojas is to the body what bliss is to the mind. Ojas is the most refined product of digestion, and brings a healthy radiance to the skin. *Charaka Samhita* explains that ojas makes the skin soft but firm, sweet-smelling, and of good color. Other signs of ojas are a balanced, blissful personality, a refined intellect, and a flowing heart. Ojas nourishes the experience of bliss in the mind and body.

Ojas is the opposite of ama, the toxic waste product of digestion. All of Maharishi Vedic Medicine's programs, therapies, and recommendations are designed to generate and maintain ojas in the body. While ama blocks the flow of biological intelligence, ojas creates a smooth, frictionless flow to every cell, leading to more integrated functioning of mind, memory, speech, and action.

When ojas is lively, immunity is high and the mind and body function as an integrated whole.

Maharishi Vedic Medicine emphasizes ojas both for its role in preventing disease and for its great significance in the evolution of human life and consciousness. It provides a lively link between the abstract field of pure consciousness and the physical matter of the body, promoting higher states of consciousness. With the full enlivenment of ojas, a fully awake consciousness blossoms, and sickness and suffering get eliminated at their basis.

Ojas is always present in the body to some degree. Ojas is located in the heart, where it sustains life itself. It also circulates throughout the body. The healthier you are, the more ojas you produce. The healthier the foods you eat, the better your digestion. Then you produce more ojas, which circulates throughout your body creating better health, happiness, and immunity from disease. The apple you eat goes through many transformations until it becomes ojas and, ultimately, consciousness itself.

Ojas plays a special role during pregnancy, because the mother provides ojas for her baby. The *Charaka Samhita* says,

It is the ojas which keeps all the living beings
refreshed. There can be no life without ojas. Ojas
marks the beginning of the formation of the embryo.
It is the nourishing fluid from the embryo. It enters
the heart right at the stage of the [embryo's] initial
formation. Loss of ojas amounts to the loss of life itself.
It sustains the life and is located in the heart. It
constitutes the essence of all tissue elements." [23]

Because you, as the mother, are the source for ojas in your child, you'll want to eat the best possible foods and optimize your ability to digest them. The goal is to transform all your food into the very nourishing, blissful ojas. Throughout your pregnancy and postpartum period, you'll want to take care to eat the foods that have an inherent purity. These easily digestible foods enhance the formation of reproductive tissue and produce ojas. The essence of the reproductive tissue (or *shukra*, introduced in Chapter Four) is nourished by these foods, creating healthier offspring and providing rich, healthy breast milk.

But perhaps the most important result of ojas for an expectant mother is the feeling of well-being, of joyful, euphoric happiness, that pervades the mind and body when ojas is present. This is a state of being in love with life, of feeling that you occupy the right place in the world, of being in tune with nature. This feeling of bliss, the emotional experience of ojas, is the state of pure love. What could be more nourishing to your child than this?

Easily Digestible (Sattvic) Foods

There are a few foods that are especially nourishing to expectant mothers, which are called *sattvic*, meaning "pure." These ojas-producing foods include milk, butter, ghee, fresh fruits, fresh fruit juices, rice, wheat, sesame seeds, split mung beans, fresh coconut (not dried), oranges, dates, raisins, blanched almonds, and raw honey. These foods are known to produce ojas.

Milk is an especially sattvic food that is nourishing to you and your baby. The best way to prepare milk is to boil it first. This makes it more digestible. Adding a little cardamom or turmeric also adds to its digestibility. Please note that milk doesn't digest well if you drink it with a full meal, especially one including the salty and sour tastes, since these foods cause the milk to curdle. It's better to drink milk alone as a snack or with other sweet-tasting foods, such as ghee, rice, and wheat. Many mothers who have trouble drinking milk are able to digest it easily after trying these recommendations.

Ghee is also a highly sattvic and nourishing food for expectant mothers. *Charaka Samhita* says that unctuous food (i.e., food prepared with healthy oils, such as ghee or olive oil) is not only delicious, but it promotes the subtle power of digestion, gets digested quickly, helps in the downward movement of Apana Vata, enhances the senses, promotes strength, and brings out the brightness of complexion.[24] Because its molecular structure differs from most animal fats, ghee is much safer and more nourishing.[25] Recent studies have found that, if taken in moderation, ghee does not raise cholesterol.[26] Ghee is highly prized in Maharishi Vedic Medicine, because it increases agni and creates ojas.

You can make ghee* by simmering sweet (unsalted) butter until the milk solids sink to the bottom. What is left is a clear, golden cooking oil that doesn't burn while heated. Pour that through cheese cloth or a fine-mesh strainer into a clean, dry jar, and store it at room temperature. Do not refrigerate. It will remain good for months as a soft solid that can be spread on toast and melted over vegetables.

---

* You can make ghee at home, buy it from an Indian grocery store, or see Appendix C to order.

Foods to Avoid

You'll want to avoid foods that are not easily digested, because they produce ama instead of ojas. These are called *tamasic* foods in the Vedic texts. These hard-to-digest foods include meat, poultry, fish, eggs, alcohol, aged cheeses, mushrooms, peanuts, fermented foods, leftovers, processed foods, excessive amounts of sour and salty foods, and vinegar.

Onions and garlic are also considered tamasic, and are discouraged for pregnant women by the Vedic texts because hot, spicy, or sharp tastes may promote bleeding or contribute to miscarriages. Many women develop an aversion to onions and garlic when they are pregnant, which is the body's signal to avoid these foods at this time.

In general a vegetarian diet is lighter and easier to digest than a non-vegetarian diet, and you can get plenty of protein from legumes and dairy products, even during pregnancy. Of course, if you are not yet a vegetarian, pregnancy is not the time to make dramatic changes in your diet by stopping eating meat. However, you may want to see if you feel like eating less red meat. You can still get enough protein from chicken or fish, and although harder to digest than vegetarian foods, they are still more digestible and healthier for your baby than red meat. Most of my patients who are pregnant find that the diet recommended by Maharishi Vedic Medicine is both easy to digest and extremely nourishing.

Amy gave birth to the oldest of her three boys when she was 39. *"At that time I didn't know about the Maharishi Vedic Approach to Health,"* she says. *"I ate like a Trojan and strained to consume the recommended seventy grams of protein a day, which is almost impossible to do if you're a vegetarian. I remember lying on my bed and moaning to my husband that I just couldn't do it, I felt bloated. I also had terrible gas pains, which is common in pregnancy because your stomach gets compressed and the baby's kicking also disturbs digestion. I put on fabulous amounts of weight, which was difficult to lose later, and my son was huge at birth—weighing ten and one-quarter pounds.*

"With my second child, I consulted a physician trained in Maharishi Vedic Medicine and followed the diet for pregnancy, which is so nourishing yet light and easy to digest. I felt satisfied after each meal but not bloated. I also followed the recommendations for improving digestion (not overeating, sitting down while I ate, etc.) and my digestion was great—no gas pains at all. So the diet and the guidelines for improving digestion made me feel much more comfortable and healthy throughout. I ate enough protein and gained a normal amount of weight. My son was born a healthy eight pounds."

Prenatal Herbal Supplements

Besides giving dietary advice for pregnancy, the Vedic texts describe herbal supplements for the pregnant woman to help nourish the fetus. For instance, *Sushruta Samhita* contains a special chapter which prescribes different foods and herbs for each month of pregnancy, as the nutritional needs of the fetus change as it develops. The kidneys, for instance, are developing at a certain time and the heart at another time, and different nutrients are needed to support the growth of different organs.

Traditionally, special herbal compounds called *rasayanas* are routinely prescribed to pregnant women to help with the well-being and growth of the fetus. Rasayanas are intended to have a strengthening and rejuvenating effect, and to increase ojas in the mother and child. An entire regimen of rasayanas, herbal decoctions, and flavorings called *churnas* are started on day one of pregnancy to strengthen both mother and baby and prevent complications. These different herbal preparations and rasayanas also promote the development of different organs. Unfortunately, many of these rasayanas and herbal preparations are not yet available in the United States due to federal regulations.

Some modern researchers, including epidemiologist Dr. David

J. P. Barker, who pioneered in the field, feel that low birth weight (except in premature babies or twins) may be linked to disease later in life. The theory is that if the fetus is undernourished at critical times during pregnancy, then the nutrients will be diverted from certain organs to more important areas, such as the brain. The organ that is being formed at that time will be damaged. For instance, the kidneys are being formed in the thirty-second and thirty-third weeks. After that, no new kidney cells are made. In this way, fluctuations in the flow of nutrition may permanently change the structure of the heart, liver, kidneys, blood vessels, and more. It appears that diseases such as strokes, diabetes, high blood pressure, and heart disease may have their origins in the womb.[27]

The Vedic seers also saw this connection, which is why so much emphasis is placed on nourishing the organs of the fetus with special food supplements as they are developing.

That's also why it's important to eat a balanced diet and to respond to the mother's cravings during pregnancy, since fulfilling these cravings fulfills the nutritional and developmental needs of the infant (a point also understood by modern obstetrics).

Summary

Eating right is more important when you are pregnant, because your baby's sole means of nourishment comes from you. By eating foods of all six tastes, you can bring greater balance to your diet. And you can follow simple guidelines for helping your digestion run smoothly. Then your body can extract the greatest nutritional value from your food—and thus give the most nourishment to your baby.

"A pregnant woman is to be treated very cautiously, as if one is walking with a pot full of oil in hand without letting a drop fall."   —*Charaka Samhita*[28]

"From [the time of conception] onwards, a pregnant woman should never indulge in physical exertion, over-eating, fasting, day sleeping, keeping awake at night, grief, riding on bicycles, fear, squatting, untimely blood letting, procedures of purification, and sexual intercourse, and should never suppress the calls of nature (i.e., urination, etc.)."
     —*Sushruta Samhita*[29]

CHAPTER SEVEN

Daily Routine and Exercise

During your pregnancy, you will need a lot more rest. Even though you'll probably be busy getting ready for the baby, and will have all kinds of projects and plans, it's important to remember that staying rested will help your baby much more than wallpapering the nursery.

Resting more is especially important during the first two months and the last two months of pregnancy. You may find you feel best when you go to bed earlier, as early as eight or nine o'clock. The deep rest from practicing the Transcendental Meditation program twice a day will also revitalize and energize you. As your pregnancy progresses, you'll probably want to get off your feet and put your legs up at intervals. The rule is: rest before you are tired. Remember, your body already has an extra load to carry. Over-exerting yourself to the point of exhaustion can be harmful to you and your baby.

Maintaining a daily routine in tune with nature's rhythms is an important aspect of Maharishi Vedic Medicine, called *dinacharya*. In this chapter you will learn some of the principles for harnessing the energy of nature in your own life—by eating, sleeping and acting in tune with natural rhythms.

Karen, age 33, a mother of two boys, says, *"I took a lot of extra rest with my first child. I was able to go to bed early. It was very clear, the effects of*

being on a restful routine. I practiced the Transcendental Meditation tech-
nique, and after each meditation I felt much better, more energetic, and happy.
I would sleep a lot more during meditation than usual, but I could feel the
baby more when I meditated, clearly felt his presence inside me."

What Are the Rhythms of Nature?

Everyone's had them—the kind of day when you wake up fresh
and alert, and you have a special feeling that everything will go
your way. And it does—you just seem to be in the right place at
the right time. Instead of struggling to get everything done,
you're filled with abundant energy and accomplish your work easily. And at the end of the day, instead of feeling fatigued, you drift
off to sleep feeling satisfied and fulfilled.

This kind of perfect day, when you feel in tune with nature,
doesn't have to be a rare experience. If you can align your daily
routine to nature's rhythms you can enjoy deeper sleep, more dy-
namic activity, and better health the year 'round.

One of the most obvious cycles of nature is expressed in the
change of seasons. As you probably remember from your grade
school science class, the Earth revolves around the sun in a cycle
of 365¼ days. Because the Earth's axis is tilted, parts of the globe
are tilted toward the sun at certain times of the year, creating the
warmer summer season. At other times they are tilted away from
the sun, creating the colder winter season.

Another important cycle is the circadian rhythm—a twenty-
four-hour cycle that takes place as the Earth rotates on its axis.
This alteration of light and darkness causes many changes in your
body, and you naturally feel like sleeping when it's dark and being
alert when it's light. So your sleep-wakefulness cycle is one of
these circadian rhythms.

There are other powerful cycles of nature, such as the combined cycles of the moon and sun which move the vast ocean in
the rhythm of the tides, and the moon's changing phases as it

revolves around the Earth.

All of these have a powerful effect on your body. In fact, an entire branch of modern medicine is now emerging, called behavioral chronobiology, which studies the changes in hormone levels and other vital functions during different phases of these cycles. Recent research shows that many neurological and endocrine functions follow the twenty-four-hour circadian cycle, including temperature fluctuations, hormone and enzyme functions, electrolyte excretion, etc. Certain medicines create widely varying results depending on what time of day they are administered.

Maharishi Vedic Medicine recognizes that the vital force of every cell in your body ebbs and flows in the rhythms of nature. But to take advantage of these cycles, you need first to understand that at their basis lie the three fundamental rhythms of Vata, Pitta, and Kapha.

The Three Basic Rhythms of Vata, Pitta, and Kapha

You'll remember from Chapter Three that the three doshas, Vata, Pitta, and Kapha, are the governing principles of your body and all of nature. They are the forces that shape the cycles we have been talking about.

Not only do the three doshas express themselves in different seasons (Vata in the cold and dry winter, Kapha in the cool and wet spring, and Pitta in the hot and humid summer), but they also govern different times of the day. Every twenty-four-hour period contains two full cycles of these three.

In the early evening, when darkness is falling, the wild birds and animals become less active and prepare for sleep. As the day ends, all of nature seems to slow down, and there is a heavier, quieter feeling in the air. This corresponds to Kapha dosha, which is heavy and slow by nature. Contrast this with sunrise, when the birds literally burst into song, reflecting the active, vital feeling of the new day. This time of day reflects the qualities of Vata dosha, which is active, moving, and full of vitality. And as the sun rises high in the sky at the noon hour, the hot Pitta dosha is more active, and our digestion is at its strongest.

Daily Rhythms of Vata, Pitta, and Kapha

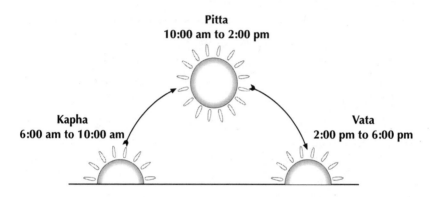

Pitta
10:00 am to 2:00 pm

Kapha
6:00 am to 10:00 am

Vata
2:00 pm to 6:00 pm

CYCLE ONE—FROM DAWN TO DUSK

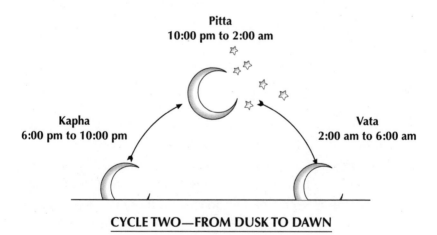

Pitta
10:00 pm to 2:00 am

Kapha
6:00 pm to 10:00 pm

Vata
2:00 am to 6:00 am

CYCLE TWO—FROM DUSK TO DAWN

How to Create an Optimal Daily Routine

When to wake up, when to sleep, when to eat—there is an ideal time of day for all important functions, based on these cycles of Vata, Pitta and Kapha. If you follow your body's natural rhythms, you'll naturally fall asleep faster, digest your food more thoroughly, and feel energetic throughout the day.

Just as it's easier to flow with the current of the river, following the routine is actually quite easy, because your body wants to follow its natural rhythms. There are two crucial times in your routine: going to bed early and waking up early. Let's look at these.

Early to Bed: How you feel when you wake up in the morning really depends on what time you went to bed. The evening routine is designed to allow your body to fall asleep quickly and to sleep deeply. According to Maharishi Vedic Medicine, "sleep is the nurse of all living beings." Because your body can heal itself better when it gets enough rest, in the Maharishi Vedic Approach to Health, sleep is one of the three pillars of health.

Unfortunately, an astounding fifty million Americans complain of insomnia. Insomnia is most commonly caused by a disturbance in Vata dosha. When Vata is out of balance, your mind can be so busy and your body so keyed up that you just can't fall asleep.

People with Vata disorders tend to keep irregular habits, eating at different times of the night or day, and going to bed at all hours. Such a haphazard daily schedule is the worst thing for treating Vata dosha. In fact, being out of tune with nature's daily rhythms may be causing insomnia in many people who artificially extend the daylight hours with electric lights. For Americans of an earlier century, it was natural to go to bed when it got dark.

Why is it better to fall asleep earlier? Because the early evening is the Kapha time of day (6:00 p.m. to 10:00 p.m.). This is when the heavier, duller qualities of Kapha dosha predominate, which are conducive to sleep. So, if you fall asleep during this Kapha cycle in the early evening, your sleep will come more easily and will have more of the heavy, slow, stable quality of Kapha dosha.

Modern research concurs that sleep becomes lighter and lighter as dawn approaches. During the heavier sleep, called NonRapid Eye Movement Sleep (NREM), your body's self-repair healing mechanisms are revitalized. During the lighter, Rapid Eye Movement Sleep (REM), you dream more and release stress and tension.

The deepest, nonREM slumber occurs within twenty minutes of falling asleep, and is interrupted about ninety minutes later by a five-to-ten minute round of REM-type sleep. For the rest of the night, you alternate between the two types of sleep in ninety-minute cycles, with your nonREM sleep becoming shorter and less deep and the lighter REM cycles becoming longer.

Unfortunately, most people postpone going to bed and end up trying to fall asleep during the Pitta cycle, between 10:00 p.m. and 2:00 a.m. Sleep during this time takes on more of the qualities of Pitta dosha. Pitta dosha creates a lighter, sharper, more active quality in your body and mind at this time. If you go to sleep then, you may toss and turn all night. Also, the Pitta time of night is needed by your body for repair, rejuvenation, and clearing the body's channels of ama. If you stay up late, you tend to get hungry and eat during this Pitta time, which does not allow your digestive system to rest and cleanse itself, and can create more ama in the system.

In other words, you can spend the same amount of time asleep, but it won't be the same sweet, deep sleep as if you go to bed during the Kapha cycle. You'll probably find that eight hours starting at 9:30 is twice as restful as eight hours starting at 2:00 a.m.

Remember to eat a light meal in the evening, preferably before 8:00 p.m. As we discussed in Chapter Six, eating light at night is better for digestion. You'll also find that you sleep better when you eat light. Save the evening hours for quieter, more relaxing activities. Even watching TV before bed can aggravate Vata and disturb your sleep. If you must watch TV, try to turn it off before 9:00 p.m. Listening to soothing music, visiting with friends, and spending time with your children are recommended evening activities.

And Early to Rise: Often people feel groggy in the morning and continue to feel groggy all day. In fact, most people probably think it's normal to wake up feeling tired. But in many cases, this may be due to unnatural sleep habits. As you start to follow the daily routine of early to bed and early to rise, and begin to experience more balance in your mind and body, you'll find yourself waking up feeling lighter and more buoyant.

Aside from going to bed early and getting enough sleep, it is equally important that you get up early, before 6:00 a.m., when the morning Kapha cycle starts. While the evening Kapha cycle is optimum for falling asleep, the morning Kapha cycle (from 6:00 a.m. to 10:00 a.m.) is not a good time to be sleeping. If you wake up during the Kapha cycle in the morning, your system gets suffused with the dull, slow, heavy qualities of Kapha—making you feel dull and tired throughout the day.

That's why Maharishi Vedic Medicine recommends that you wake up with the birds (before 6:00 a.m.), during the morning Vata cycle. Then you'll feel more of the Vata qualities (energy, vitality, alertness) throughout the day.

Getting up early and at the same time every day, regardless of what time you went to bed the night before, is one of the most important steps to putting yourself in tune with nature's rhythms. The logic for this is simple—if you get up consistently early, over a few days or weeks you will start to feel sleepy earlier in the evening.

Avoiding Daytime Sleep During Pregnancy

Even though rest is the most important component of a smooth pregnancy, it's interesting that daytime naps are not recommended in Maharishi Vedic Medicine. This is because the vital channels of the body get clogged when you sleep during the day, leaving you feeling lethargic and dull. Daytime sleep also aggravates all three doshas, throwing the body out of balance. That's why it's better to get a good night's sleep by going to bed early. Then you will enjoy the full benefit of nature's vitality by staying in tune with natural rhythms.

There are times when it's fine to sleep during the day, of course, such as when you're sick, and when you're recovering from travel. Also, young children and the elderly need to nap. And during the summer the body's channels stay open because of the heat, so then it is fine to sleep during the day.

The best way to rest during the day is to practice the Transcendental Meditation technique twice a day. This gives you a quality of rest that leaves your mind clear and fresh.

⋰ MORE RELAXED PHYSIOLOGY ⋱

Physiological Indicators of Deep Rest
Through the *Transcendental Meditation* Technique

A meta-analysis found that the Transcendental Meditation technique produced a significant decrease in basal skin conductance compared to eyes-closed rest, indicating profound relaxation. Deep rest and relaxation were also indicated by similarly greater decreases in respiration rates and plasma lactate.

References: 1. M.C. Dillbeck and D.W. Orme-Johnson, "Physiological Differences between Transcendental Meditation and Rest," *American Psychologist*, 42 (1987), pp. 879-881.
2. R.K. Wallace, "Physiological Effects of Transcendental Meditation," *Science*, 167 (1970), pp. 1751-1754.
3. R.K. Wallace, et al., "A Wakeful Hypometabolic Physiologic State," *American Journal of Physiology*, 221 (1971), pp. 795-799.

The Daily Routine

WAKE-UP ROUTINE

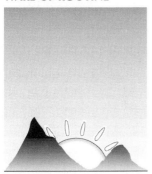

- Wake up early, before 6:00 a.m.
- Evacuate bowels and bladder.
- Brush your teeth and scrape your tongue.
- Give yourself an *abhyanga* (oil massage).
- Bathe or shower.
- Do Yoga asanas (neuromuscular integration exercises) and breathing techniques.
- Practice the Transcendental Meditation technique.
- Exercise.
- Eat a light breakfast.

MIDDAY ROUTINE

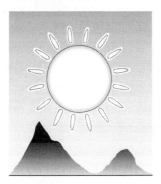

- Work or study.
- Eat your largest meal between 12:00 noon and 1:00 p.m.
- Take a brief walk to aid digestion.
- Work or study.

NIGHTTIME ROUTINE

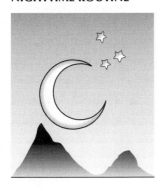

- Do Yoga asanas and breathing techniques in the late afternoon or early evening.
- Practice the Transcendental Meditation technique.
- Eat an early, light dinner.
- Take a brief walk to aid digestion.
- Enjoy light, relaxing activities.
- Go to sleep before 10:00 p.m.

Daily Oil Massage for Pregnancy

A special full-body self-massage called *abhyanga* is a key element of the daily routine, and is especially healthy in pregnancy. Most people find this to be a relaxing and energizing way to start the day. Massaging your body with warm sesame oil will soothe Vata dosha, which you'll remember has light, cold and dry qualities. Vata dosha is the main dosha that goes out of balance from stress, and it can also cause fatigue. If you remember, Vata also plays a special role during pregnancy, and you can avoid many of the discomforts of pregnancy by balancing Vata. Abhyanga also promotes increased strength and immunity.

The daily abhyanga helps energize and stimulate all the organs of the body, which makes it a gentle way to wake yourself up and dissolve the lethargy of the previous night's sleep. Abhyanga increases circulation throughout the body, loosening and removing impurities—not to mention how it cleanses and tones the skin. Many expectant mothers report that the daily massage helps to keep their skin flexible and minimizes stretch marks. You can receive instruction in abhyanga from a physician/practitioner trained in Maharishi Vedic Medicine.

Guidelines for Abhyanga:

1. Use cured sesame oil for the massage—ideally unprocessed, cold-pressed sesame oil, available at health food stores.* To cure the oil, place up to one quart of it in a saucepan and heat it to the boiling temperature of *water*. (It's important to realize that you don't need to boil the *oil*, as that could be dangerous.) Use a candy thermometer to monitor the heat constantly. **As the oil begins to heat, the temperature will begin to rise more quickly, so watch it very carefully.** Once it reaches 212 degrees, the oil is cured and you should immediately remove it from the heat

---

* See Appendix C to order.

and place it on a cool surface, such as in your sink or on a hot pad on your countertop. **Be very careful to follow safety precautions** (your kitchen should naturally be equipped with a fire extinguisher), **and never leave the oil on the stove while you are out of the room.** The whole process takes only about five minutes, and you can cure enough to last for several weeks.

2. Warm the oil slightly before the massage. An easy way to do this is to place a small quantity of cured oil in a fliptop plastic container and immerse it in warm water for a few minutes, or in a baby bottle warmer.

3. In general, use an open palm rather than your fingertips. Use long strokes on the long bones of the body and circular strokes on the joints.

4. Apply a light covering of oil to each part of the body before massaging it.

5. Be very gentle when massaging your abdomen—you don't need to rub, but just apply oil lightly.

6. In the eighth and ninth months, be sure to not to skip your breasts. The oil massage is a good preparation for nursing.

Massage your head, ears, and face first. Using a circular motion, massage the top, sides, and back of the head with both hands. Gently massage the outer ears.

Circle the temples and cheeks. Stroke across the forehead. Stroke across the upper lip and chin.

Next massage the front and back of the neck, using horizontal strokes back and forth. Be gentle over the windpipe.

Massage each arm separately. Circle the shoulder, use long strokes back and forth on the upper arm, circle the elbow, and use long strokes back and forth on the lower arm. Circle the wrist. Massage the palm of the hand and the back of the hand, then pull each finger gently.

The chest and abdomen are next. Make circles on the chest with both hands, using very gentle, circular motion over the heart. Be very gentle on the abdomen, using a clockwise motion (to follow the natural direction of the elimination system).

On the back, use long strokes to massage up and down the spine and back (as far as you can reach).

Legs are similar to arms. Massage each leg separately, and use long strokes on the upper leg, circular strokes on the knee, and long strokes on the calf. Circle the ankles.

The feet are last, but you'll want to spend more time here. Massage back and forth on the Achilles' tendon, heel, and top of the foot. Use the palm of the hand to stroke lengthwise on the sole of the foot. Gently pull the toes.

After your abhyanga, you'll want to rinse off the sesame oil in a warm bath. Bathing in warm water also helps open the channels of circulation and allows the impurities that have been loosened through the massage to flow out into the digestive tract. If you cannot take a bath, try a warm shower.

You may think you are too busy to add the abhyanga to your daily routine, but the mothers who do find that the benefits far outweigh any inconvenience.

Sally, a mother who conceived unexpectedly at age forty-one, says, *"I did the abhyanga every day of my pregnancy. With going to school full-time, working, and moving to a big city after nine years in a small town, there was a lot more stress in my life. I found that doing the oil massage was what really kept me in my center point. Once in a while I had to skip it just because of my schedule, but on those days I felt vulnerable and off. It seemed to give me a protective armor, so to speak—and a really smooth, clear experience in activity. I suspect it was very relaxing for my baby as well. Everything went so well with the pregnancy and birth—and now I'm enjoying my healthy baby girl."*

How Much Exercise During Pregnancy?

Maharishi Vedic Medicine emphasizes that you should take every precaution to avoid straining your abdomen, lifting heavy objects, etc., and to avoid any jolting, sharp movements. So doing sit-ups would not be good, because they strain the abdomen, and sports involving jumping, jogging, and running would be too jarring.

Walking and swimming are probably the ideal forms of exercise, especially if done in the morning. And of course, it's healthy to get fresh air every day. It's good to be active, and the more active you are the easier your labor will be.

One of the most beneficial exercises during pregnancy is a specific series of gentle bending postures. These neuromuscular integration exercises are known as *Yoga asanas. Asana* means "established," referring to being established in pure consciousness—the goal of all the approaches of Maharishi Vedic Medicine (see Chapter Two). Asanas are known to increase circulation, improve mind-body coordination, and create both flexibility and strength. Traditionally, there are different postures to purify and strengthen the major glands, organs, and systems of the body. Asanas help dissolve much of the gross fatigue and stress in the body and thus are a valuable preparation for meditation.

For pregnant women, Yoga asanas can help relax, tone, strengthen, rejuvenate, and purify the body. They also help calm the emotions, and create a serene, settled feeling of well-being. Because asanas are so simple to do, they are an ideal exercise for busy mothers-to-be. Properly performed, they are safe and gentle, never jarring or taxing to the mother. There are many specific asanas for all stages of giving birth, including pregnancy, preparation for childbirth, and postpartum.

If you would like to learn Yoga asanas, you can ask your physician/practitioner for instructions. There are also special Maharishi Yoga[SM] courses offered through Maharishi Vedic Universities and Schools.*

If you are already accustomed to doing asanas, talk to your ob-

---

* See Appendix C.

stetrician to make sure you should continue doing them during pregnancy. Usually, you can follow your usual asana routine during the first three months, although you'll want to avoid any positions that invert the uterus, such as headstands (which Maharishi Vedic Medicine discourages anyway), shoulder stands, or the "plow." From three to six months, you'll need to modify your routine to accommodate your expanding uterus. Any positions causing strain or discomfort should be eliminated—such as the "cobra," "locust," or any position which involves lying on or putting pressure on your abdomen. After the sixth month, you will probably want to discontinue the asanas, unless your obstetrician recommends that you stop earlier or continue certain postures longer.

If you are accustomed to lots of physical exercise, the most important thing is never to strain, and to consult your obstetrician to make sure your exercise level is safe for your baby.

Terri, a 31-year-old physical education teacher who continued teaching until six weeks before delivery, recalls her pregnancy. *"The first instruction I followed was to listen to my body. And of course, to make sure I was protecting my baby, I never did any activity that would invert the uterus or cramp the stomach. I didn't do sit-ups, and I never wore clothing that was binding around the waist. But that left me a lot of latitude. I was able to walk, so I walked to school twice a day. I didn't run any more because I didn't want to jar the baby. I did whatever was comfortable, and if I felt any discomfort, I just pulled back. I used principles of moderation."*

Summary

Resting is important during pregnancy, as your body needs more rest. It's also important to get fresh air and mild exercise every day. If you follow a daily routine in tune with nature's rhythms, you'll feel more energetic throughout the day.

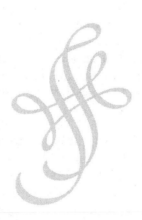

"The pregnant woman from the first day [of conception] should always remain in a happy mood, be clean, wear ornaments, dress in white clothes, and be engaged in prayers for peace, good deeds, and worship of God."   —*Sushruta Samhita*[30]

"The pregnant woman should avoid foul odors, bad scenes, and stories that might disturb mental equilibrium. She should not eat dry, stale, rotten, or fermented food …. She should avoid feelings of anger and fear, talking loudly and all other things that could be detrimental to the growth of the fetus ….
Neither should she fatigue her body.

"Her seat and bed should be covered with soft clothes, should not be very high and should be well supported and comfortable. She should be given to eat palatable, liquid, sweet, and demulcent foods mixed with appetizing herbs. This should be the general way of living until delivery takes place."
          —*Sushruta Samhita*[31]

CHAPTER EIGHT

Staying Happy During Pregnancy

Pregnancy is a time to pamper yourself, get lots of rest, and above all, be happy. It cannot be emphasized enough how important this is. Just as your thoughts and feelings affect your own physical body, everything that you think, hear, feel, and do will affect your baby.

This does not mean that if you have temporary moments of fear or anger that your unborn child will suffer. However, if you are feeling waves of love toward your child, and you and your husband are eagerly awaiting the birth, your child will thrive mentally and physically on that love.

In one research study, it was found that maternal attitude was by far the most important factor in determining a child's emotional and physical well-being.[32] If a mother has a positive feeling about her baby and about childbearing, she is much more likely to give birth to a healthy, emotionally well-adjusted child.

For that reason, pregnancy is not the time to plan big changes, such as moving. In one recent study, 79 percent of the women interviewed said that they were planning to move into a bigger home now that they were expecting a baby. Yet the anxiety, disorientation, and exhaustion caused by a move can actually delay the mother's bonding with her baby after birth, or contribute to postpartum depression.[33]

In the Vedic tradition, women are pampered during pregnancy. While growing up in India, I observed great pride in the family when a new member was expected. Everyone knows that it's important to keep the mother happy, so nearly every day a neighbor or friend or relative will bring the pregnant woman something special, some sweets or a gift. The family always cooks special foods for the pregnant woman—to always make sure she gets what she likes. It's part of the tradition to make special sweets for her cravings and for her needs. It is ingrained in the culture that if the woman is not happy, the baby will not be happy. So the mother is encouraged to rest more during pregnancy. Usually the husband takes on more household responsibilities, and if the couple is living with the in-laws, they help out, too.

The Role of the Father

Your husband has a special role to play during your pregnancy—keeping you as contented and comfortable as possible! It's a time for your husband to give you lots of attention and to spend extra time with you both morning and evening. It's important to spend more time alone at this time, because once the baby is born there will be fewer chances for free time together. In my practice, I try to explain to the husband that an expectant mother may be more delicate emotionally and physically. He should be especially nurturing, caring, and understanding of her needs and desires at this time.

A happy marriage is one of the major factors in determining a smooth pregnancy and healthy child. If the mother is surrounded by love and her desires are acknowledged and supported by her husband, she transmits that love to her baby.

Recent research shows that the father's relationship with the mother and his attitude toward the unborn child have a great effect on the child's mental and physical health later in life. In fact, many researchers feel that the father's attitude is a highly important factor in a healthy pregnancy, second only to the mother's.[34]

A strained marriage or relationship is considered by some researchers to be the cause of emotional and physical damage in the womb. In one study involving more than 1300 children and their families, it was found that an expectant mother in an abusive marriage has a 237 percent greater risk of giving birth to a psychologically or physically damaged child than a woman in a secure, nourishing relationship. This is even a greater risk than that caused by the mother smoking or having a severe physical illness.[34]

⋰ HEALTHIER HOME LIFE ⋱

More Ideal Family Relationships

Researchers examined two sets of families practicing the Transcendental Meditation technique. The ones practicing the TM technique for a longer time (five years or more) exhibited higher levels of psychological health than did the short-term (less than one year) meditating families, whose scores were similar to normal families. This indicates that continued practice of the TM technique helps develop more ideal family life.

Reference: M.E. Chen, "A Comparative Study of Dimensions of Healthy Functioning Between Families Practicing the TM program for Five Years or for Less than a Year," *Dissertation Abstracts International*, 45 (10) (1984), p. 3206B.

Although it is important for the husband to express his tender feelings for his wife and child by being affectionate, it's recommended to abstain from sexual intercourse during pregnancy, especially the last three months. According to *Charaka Samhita*, the parents protect the fetus from possible mental, physical, and emotional harm by abstaining during pregnancy. Intercourse can precipitate labor and cause uterine contractions. In any case, it is best to follow your obstetrician's advice.

Music Therapy

According to the Vedic texts, there are several factors that determine the state of the mental abilities of the child, including the mental faculties of the parents and the sounds or music heard repeatedly by the pregnant woman.[36] If a mother listens to uplifting, nourishing music, this will nourish her baby's intelligence.

Even plants respond differently to different kinds of music. In widely publicized research, it was found that plants tend to flourish and grow toward the speaker when soothing music is played to them, and they turn away from the speaker when rock music is played.[37] During the last thirty years, there has been an upsurge of interest in music as a means to heal the mind and body. Researchers have found that music affects the pulse rate, circulation, and blood pressure.[38, 39]

Music therapy was used in the Vedic civilization of India to create balance in the individual and society, and after that, by the Greeks and Persians. In fact, one common recommendation of Maharishi Vedic Medicine is to listen to Maharishi Gandharva Veda[SM] music, which uses melodies and rhythms of nature to attune the body to the specific laws of nature operating at certain times of the day. There are actually different musical compositions (called *ragas*) for twelve different time periods during the day. This is because the frequencies of nature are different at different times in the day—for example, the frequencies in the morning are different from those operating at night. Playing Maharishi Gandharva Veda music helps you to attune yourself to these subtle shifts in nature, thus dissolving stress, disharmony, and fatigue.

Another aspect of Maharishi Vedic Medicine uses "primordial sounds," the basic impulses of nature's intelligence in the Veda and the Vedic Literature, to restore and maintain optimal health. These sounds have specific wave characteristics that are said to rejuvenate the body and restore balance to the system.

In a recently published study it was found that the primordial sounds known as *Sama Veda* significantly decreased growth of human tumor cell lines (for lung, colon, brain, breast, and skin cancer) in test-tube cultures. When exposed to hard rock music, the cancer cells grew significantly. It appears that the low, sooth-ing sounds of Sama Veda help the growth of normal cells.[40]

You can imagine that the cells forming your new baby's body could be similarly affected. That's why you want to expose your-self only to the most uplifting music and sounds. It's also a great way to get extra rest and to rejuvenate while you're pregnant. You can take five or ten minutes off from work to close your eyes, put up your feet and listen to primordial sounds of the Veda or Maharishi Gandharva Veda music. You can also play these in your home—even if you're not always there to hear them—to create a peaceful, harmonious atmosphere.*

Baby Showers

The baby's senses develop during the third month, which is when you will probably start experiencing food cravings and un-usual desires. As I mentioned in Chapter Five, these are the de-sires of the baby and should be fulfilled. If you try to suppress these desires, it puts a strain on the baby.

When I was growing up in India, my family followed the Vedic custom of giving baby showers for the pregnant women of the family. From the third month of pregnancy on, friends and family traditionally hold a different baby shower each month to cel-ebrate the development of each of the five senses in the unborn child. The first shower celebrates the developing sense of sight, so gifts include objects that are beautiful to look at. The second shower celebrates the sense of taste, so many delicious foods are served. As the sense of hearing develops, the third shower fea-tures melodious and soothing music. The shower celebrating the sense of smell includes many delightful aromas. Finally, in the last shower, clothing and gold are given to celebrate the sense of touch. These showers create a loving and nourishing environ-

---

* See Appendix C to order Gandharva Veda Music® tapes or CDs.

ment in which the mother and baby can flourish in health and happiness.

Showers such as these also point out the role of the extended family in many cultures. In most traditional cultures around the world, the pregnant woman is never left alone, but is surrounded by female relatives and friends at all times. While you may not have a mother or sister living with you, it's a good idea when you're pregnant to spend more time with mothers of young children, especially if this is your first child.

Experienced mothers can give you advice and reassurance if you ever feel worried. In this way, you'll very naturally grow in confidence in your new role as a mother.

Uplifting Entertainment

Because your baby will be affected by anything that you hear, see, or feel, you will want to avoid tense, frightening movies, depressing books, and unpleasant company. You may find that you are more emotional than usual, so you'll want to protect those tender feelings and surround yourself with happy, uplifting influences.

Reading uplifting stories can have a very soothing effect, and can also help nourish your child. Stories from the ancient Vedic tradition, such as the *Ramayana* and *Mahabharata*, are filled with tales about heroes, heroines, and ideal relationships. The traditional Vedic texts used in Maharishi Vedic Medicine assert that such uplifting stories can have a beneficial effect on the character and intelligence of your child.

There is a story from the *Mahabharata*, the great epic of the Vedic Literature, which illustrates this idea. Subadhra, the wife of the virtuous and great hero Arjuna, loved to listen to his stories of great warriors while her son Abhimanyu was in the womb. When Subadhra's son was born, he already knew many secret strategies, having learned them in the womb. He became a great warrior and helped save the world from destruction.

Boris Brott, the conductor of the Hamilton, Ontario, Philharmonic Symphony Orchestra, tells of a similar experience. As a young man, he was perplexed by his ability to know certain pieces of music sight unseen. He'd be conducting a score and suddenly

---

∾ INNER HAPPINESS ∾

**Increased Self-Actualization
Through the *Transcendental Meditation* Technique**

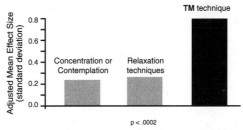

p < .0002

Statistical meta-analysis of all available studies (42 independent outcomes) indicated that the effect of the Transcendental Meditation program on increasing self-actualization is much greater then concentration, contemplation, or relaxation techniques. Self-actualization refers to realizing more of one's inner potential, expressed in every area of life: integration and stability of personality, self-regard, emotional maturity, capacity for warm interpersonal relationships, and adaptive response to challenges.

Reference: C.N. Alexander, M. Rainforth and P. Gelderloos, "TM, Self-Actualization, and Psychological Health: A Conceptual Overview and Statistical Meta-Analysis," *Journal of Social Behavior and Personality*, 6 (1991), pp. 189-247.

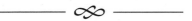

Orientation Towards Positive Values

In three studies of college students, practitioners of the Transcendental Meditation and TM-Sidhi programs exhibited more positive attitudes and perceptions than did controls, in terms of memory, recognition threshhold, and interpersonal appraisal.

Reference: P. Gelderloos, P.H. Goddard III, H.H.B. Ahlstrom, and R. Jacoby, "Cognitive Orientation Toward Positive Values in Advanced Participants of the TM and TM-Sidhi Program," *Perceptual and Motor Skills*, 64 (1987) pp. 1003-1012.

---

the cello line would jump out at him—he'd know the melody before he even turned the page. He mentioned this to his mother, who was a cellist. When he told her which cello pieces he spontaneously knew, she identified them as ones she had played while he was in the womb.[41]

Creating Happiness Within

You can't gain happiness by pretending to be happy. But you can cultivate inner happiness by becoming stronger mentally, physically, and emotionally. By providing deep rest and alleviating stress, practicing the Transcendental Meditation technique creates a state of mind that is naturally relaxed and happy. When you are happy inside, others tend to respond more positively to you, which spontaneously makes relationships—and pregnancy—easier and more fulfilling.

Summary

Research shows that your thoughts, feelings, and actions affect your unborn child. That's why your main job as a pregnant mother is to enjoy and be happy. Happy mothers produce healthy, happy babies.

PART II

Blissful Postpartum Recovery

Blissful Postpartum Recovery

Given the fact that 80 percent of American mothers experience depression after giving birth, you may not think it is possible to have a blissful postpartum. Yet that is the experience of mothers described in these chapters.

After Chapter Nine describes natural methods of delivering the baby, Chapter Ten reports the experiences of mothers throughout America today who are escaping postpartum fatigue and depression by using the remarkably simple and natural techniques of the *Maharishi Ayur-Veda* Mother and Baby program. These techniques—including massage, herbal preparations, and a special diet—turn the "baby blues" into "baby bliss." Chapter Eleven explains the causes of postpartum fatigue from a Vedic perspective, and how to avoid it. In Chapter Twelve, we describe the postpartum daily routine for rejuvenating the new mother, and in Chapter Thirteen, we cover dietary principles for postpartum and breast-feeding.

"During labor the mother should be gently massaged with warm oil on her waist, sides of chest, backs, and thighs. As a result of this, the fetus is brought downwards."   — *Charaka Samhita*[42]

"The female attendants say encouraging words as [the mother] pushes, such as 'Thanks, you have delivered a child.' This gives her relief and joy, and adds to her regaining vitality."   — *Charaka Samhita*[43]

CHAPTER NINE

Delivering Your Baby

The feeling of exhilaration a mother feels when she holds her new child in her arms for the first time can be overwhelming. "I felt that the whole universe had opened up," says Cheryl, a new mother at age 42. "I wanted to laugh and cry at once. It was the peak moment of my life."

Maharishi Vedic Medicine places great emphasis on the expectant mother's diet, routine, and emotional well-being so that the delivery will occur at the right time (i.e., not too early or late); the child will have fully developed senses and motor organs; the child will be endowed with strength, brilliant complexion, intelligence, and competence; and there will be no difficulty during the time of delivery.

It is fascinating to see how completely this system understands a subtle but fundamental principle: delivery will go better if the mother is comfortable and happy. It is even recommended that the mother be surrounded by sympathetic female companions to help her through the pain of labor. The value of such encouragement is shown in a modern research finding that labor time is shortened and mothers have a much easier time caring for and bonding with their babies if they receive sympathetic support during labor.[44]

The Vedic texts even include recommendations for arranging

the delivery room to be as uplifting and comfortable as possible. It's interesting that modern medicine is finally coming to realize that mothers need a more humane and less technological atmosphere when they deliver. In recent years in America, there has been a move away from the clinical, childbirth-as-disease view. Mothers today can enjoy giving birth in a homier "birthing room" rather than the sterile hospital delivery room of the past. In many hospitals, the birthing room is in a separate wing and is equipped with double beds. Many are designed to look like a bedroom, so the father can spend the night with his wife and baby after the birth. Mothers today can choose to have a natural birth without pain-killing drugs or medical intervention, so they and their baby can be conscious during the birth. Or they can choose to give birth in the privacy and comfort of their own home, with a mid-wife in attendance.

In this country, physicians/practitioners trained in Maharishi Vedic Medicine are not able to give recommendations for delivery (unless they are also obstetricians) due to legal reasons. You will want to rely on your obstetrician for advice. Remember that throughout the nine months of pregnancy and during delivery, it is important to check with your obstetrician before adopting any new recommendations. Here is a short description of the range of knowledge available in other countries for women who consult practitioners of Maharishi Vedic Medicine.

Diet before Delivery

After the ninth month up to the time of delivery, the pregnant woman is advised to avoid heavy foods. This is the time when the growth of the fetus has slowed dramatically, so it does not require so many nutrients to support the growth of essential organs. Lighter foods that are nourishing and easy to digest are recommended, to help balance Apana Vata (which, you may remember from Chapter Three, governs the downward flow of energy and plays a key role in childbirth) and ensure an easier birth. A special diet and very gentle cleansing procedures are also recommended to help keep the colon free of blockage as delivery approaches, since a compacted colon can block normal delivery of the fetus. The *Sushruta Samhita* says, "By regular evacuation of gas and feces, the delivery becomes easy and devoid of complications."[45]

Preparation for Delivery

Both Charaka and Sushruta give detailed descriptions of a special maternity home that should be built of aromatic woods and plastered and painted white. The room should be filled with soft bedding in light, cheerful colors. The mother enters this home for labor.

Other preparations for delivery include arranging for at least one female companion to help with the delivery along with the obstetrician or midwife.

Of course, most women today want their husbands to be with them during delivery. The husband is an essential part of the process—he usually attends childbirth classes with his wife and can coach her breathing. He offers mental and emotional support during labor. If he does not want to attend, you can have a close friend or relative come instead. Some women like to have their mother or a female friend help them in addition to their husband, because it is comforting and helpful to be attended by someone who has been through labor and knows how to give support when it is needed most.

The Vedic texts describe in detail the qualities of the attendants who care for the mother during labor. They should be elderly and be mothers of many children, thereby having valuable experience. They should be sympathetic and affectionate towards the expectant mother and be of a pleasant, agreeable disposition. Resourceful, kind-hearted by nature, cheerful and tolerant of hardships, they should have skill in the art of comforting and caring for others. The pregnant woman should not have any feeling of delicacy or embarrassment with them.

This description of qualities shows once again the importance of protecting the pregnant woman from any negative influences. She needs, above all, to be surrounded by loving, nourishing, and peaceful influences at this very sensitive time of her life.

It's interesting that two eminent scientists, H. M. Klaus and H. R. Kennel, noticed a correlation between easier labor and having a supportive, experienced female companion helping the mother at all times during the birth. After discovering this phenomenon accidentally, they went on to conduct numerous research studies, as have other scientists.

In these studies, a female companion was trained to comfort the mother through loving touch, warm eye contact, and praise. A trained attendant helped at the birth in addition to the father, who was there for emotional support, but who, in the opinion of the researchers, is not trained to give the specific kind of physical and emotional support a woman really needs during childbirth.

The results of such care are surprising. In a meta-analysis of five studies of healthy mothers with normal pregnancies who gave birth in the presence of a trained female companion, it was found that the use of Caesarean section was reduced by 50 percent, the length of labor by 25 percent, the use of oxytocin (a medication used to facilitate contractions and eventually help dilate the cervix to make room for the baby's head) by 40 percent, the need for pain medication by 30 percent, the need for forceps by 40 percent, and the requests for epidurals (local anesthetics) by 60 percent. And in addition, these mothers were able to bond much more quickly with their babies after birth, and had significantly less postpartum depression.[46]

In the words of Dr. Klaus: "Women-helping-women in labor is an ancient and widespread practice …. When, in this country, birth shifted its location from home to hospital seventy years ago, many childbirth practices that evolved over centuries were lost or altered, including birth position and companionship during labor."[47]

During Labor

The Vedic texts describe in detail the kinds of symptoms that occur with imminent labor, such as pallor in the face, a sensation of the uterus dropping, etc. When these symptoms occur, labor pains begin.

When signs and symptoms of childbirth appear, the attendants can give the mother a gentle oil massage to relax her, and can wash her body with warm water. The attendants should try to keep the mother happy with comforting words and touch.

If possible, the room should be kept quiet and dimly lit. To help relax the mother, Maharishi Gandharva Veda music can be played softly in the birthing room. Aroma therapy can help, too—especially using Vata Aroma Oil.* This blend of herb-and-flower extracts is especially designed to have a calming effect and can help soothe the new mother.

It's important to remain as relaxed as possible during labor. When the muscles are relaxed, the birth will progress more quickly and easily. If there is an absence of labor pain, then the mother should not strain to push the baby out. Straining, by itself, does not cause the baby to be born, and can exhaust the mother and even hurt the fetus.

There are several different positions recommended for labor, including lying on the back and squatting. When labor pains start and pushing is recommended, then the mother should apply strain or pressure slowly in the beginning and gradually increase it.

Ideally, the husband should stay with his wife throughout the

---

* See Appendix C to order.

delivery. He or the female attendant can offer emotional support and can gently massage her abdomen and back to comfort her. The father or a female friend can also gently massage the mother's waist, sides, back, and thighs with warm sesame oil between contractions to help ease tension. Walking between contractions also enhances the progress of labor. And deep breathing helps relieve anxiety by balancing Vata dosha, which becomes especially aggravated during childbirth.

Immediately after Delivery

In the Vedic tradition, female family and friends take turns staying with the mother and baby day and night for the first ten to twelve days following delivery. Traditionally, the mother inhales herbal powders and the birthing room is fumigated with special herbs. These help to protect the mother and baby from germs and infections, and helps balance their physiologies.

Care for the Baby: Usually after birth the baby has to be stimulated to take its first breath through the lungs. Remember that in the womb the baby used its internal breathing, and derived oxygen from the placenta. Now for the first time, he will start breathing through the lungs. Gently sprinkling water, or if that doesn't work, striking two stones near the baby's ear, is recommended to rouse the baby rather than the Western practice of spanking or slapping. Massage of the newborn, bathing, cleansing of the baby's mouth and first feeding are all part of new baby care.

Care for the Mother: As for the mother, following the delivery of the placenta, she can be given a massage with oil and ghee, followed by a sponge bath, and a drink of tea or warm milk. These measures are intended to balance Vata dosha and prevent it from accumulating in the abdominal cavity. *Sushruta Samhita* recommends decoctions of specific Vata-balancing herbs for the new mother. Then, after about three days of these light liquids, she can gradually move to heavier foods, beginning with soups or hot cereal with herbs and ghee.

The Importance of Natural Childbirth

Much research has been done on the first hour after birth, when the mother and baby can establish the precious, loving bond that will nourish them both throughout their lives. Some researchers have noticed that these first hours are a special "sensitive" period, a window of opportunity for establishing the bond of love much more easily.[48]

Maharishi Vedic Medicine recommends natural childbirth if medical conditions allow it, so that the mother and child are alert after birth and can share the precious first hours together. In most traditional cultures where birth takes place at home, this happens easily and automatically. The mother experiences a surge of joy as she lets the baby nurse for the first time just minutes after birth. And the baby experiences the warmth of the mother's body, the caress of her touch, the familiar sound of her voice, and the nourishment of his first breast-feeding.

In the following chapters, you'll learn more about the natural methods that will enhance the precious bond between mother and child—to allow the love and tenderness that every mother feels for her baby to be naturally and easily expressed.

Summary

If the mother prepares properly for a natural childbirth and is given loving support and encouragement during delivery, the birth experience can be happier and more fulfilling for mother and baby.

"If the mother is afflicted with any disease, the condition becomes either difficult of cure or incurable because all the tissue elements of her body are diminished in quantity. This is because the nutrition of the mother is utilized for the most part for the growth of the fetus. Further, her body is afflicted with emptiness because of the strain involved in labor pain and the loss of fluid and blood from the body.

"Thus the new mother should be specifically treated by the massage, bath, food, and drink prepared with herbs that alleviate germs, promote vitality, and alleviate Vata."   — *Charaka Samhita*[49]

CHAPTER TEN

Mothering the Mother

Imagine yourself the day after giving birth. You're feeling intensely elated and joyful to be a new mother. But at the same time, you feel extremely vulnerable from the fatigue of delivery—and that feeling is compounded by the overwhelming responsibility of caring for your tiny, helpless baby.

If you are a typical American mother, you probably received medical support for your pregnancy and delivery, and then were basically left on your own after birth, with only a six-week postpartum check-up to look forward to. In fact, your hospital stay was probably much shorter than your mother's when she delivered you—the average stay is now only forty-eight hours. Unlike your mother, though, you probably have no one around to help you now that the baby is born. Perhaps she lives on the other coast, and your sister is a top executive who couldn't take time out to help you even if she lived nearby. Your husband was with you during labor, but he has to go back to work after two days. And you yourself have to return to your job in just three months, fully recovered and organized.

Sound intimidating? This, unfortunately, is a typical description of postpartum care in America—mothers basically left on their own without support.

Now imagine an alternative—a way to get back on your feet

feeling in control, yourself again, in days, not weeks or months. You come home from the hospital and three days after delivery, a trained woman technician brings a massage table, fresh linens, herbalized oil, and herbal preparations to strengthen and nourish your mind and body and facilitate nursing. You finish nursing your baby and then put her to bed, allowing a family member or trusted friend to babysit for a short time.

Then the technician helps you onto the massage table for an hour of complete pampering and nurturing. She gently gives you an abhyanga (oil massage) with deliciously warm oil, infused with herbs to balance and strengthen your body. Then she tucks you into bed with fresh linens, made extra cozy with hot water bottles. She lets you rest—even fall asleep—for a while after your abhyanga and then draws you a hot bath. She also gives you herbs to help with your digestion and to promote the production of breast milk, and a special diet to help your delicate digestion start running again. After several days of this, you feel surprisingly refreshed, revitalized, ready to take on the challenge—no longer overwhelming, but instead blissful—of caring for your newborn child.

What you have just read describes the Mother and Baby program available through the Maharishi Ayur-Veda Health Centers. Based on the principles of Maharishi Vedic Medicine, this program is specifically designed to rejuvenate the mother—and to nourish and create optimal development of the new baby.

Throughout the next few chapters, we'll be describing this remarkable program and telling the story of women who have enjoyed its benefits. But perhaps you're thinking that you don't live near enough to a Maharishi Ayur-Veda Health Center to take advantage of a program like this. That's all right.

Many women have been able to follow the principles described in this chapter at home after consulting a physician/practitioner trained in Maharishi Vedic Medicine. Instead of having a technician come to your home to administer the abhyanga, you can learn how to give one to yourself. You can also follow a special postpartum diet, and take Maharishi Ayur-Veda herbal compounds to rejuvenate and restore balance. Thousands of women have received enormous benefits from doing this.

So when we talk about the Mother and Baby program, we mean consulting a physician/practitioner and following some simple recommendations.

A Description of the Mother and Baby Program

Childbirth presents a dilemma. When a woman gives birth, she experiences intense, tender love for her helpless new baby. But at the same time, the fatigue and discomfort that many women experience after giving birth constitute one of life's most difficult challenges.

The Mother and Baby program is designed to help the mother recover from the strain of pregnancy and childbirth as quickly as possible. Because pregnancy and delivery drastically alter the mother's natural balance of Vata, Pitta, and Kapha, she may feel much weaker and more vulnerable than ever before. At the same time, she will need to have the stamina and energy to care for a new baby around the clock. The resulting imbalances have both physical and mental effects, and many women in America experience varying degrees of postpartum depression. (In the next chapter, we will go more deeply into the causes and treatment of postpartum depression and "baby blues.")

Your rate of recovery depends on how quickly you can bring your body into a state of balance. The unique contribution of the Mother and Baby program is that it focuses on "mothering the mother." It provides the kind of intensive nourishment that you need at this delicate time to rejuvenate your body. And when your own physical and emotional needs are taken care of, you can do your primary job with joy and ease—nourishing and loving your new baby. The whole purpose is to keep the tender feeling of love growing throughout the postpartum period.

> ## The Mother and Baby program includes
>
> - Daily abhyanga (either self-given or administered by trained technicians) to rejuvenate the body after the exhaustion of giving birth.
> - Warm baths to allow impurities to flow out and to balance the doshas.
> - A special postpartum diet, designed especially for the new mother, to nourish and strengthen her.
> - Maharishi Ayur-Veda herbal compounds to improve the quality and quantity of breast milk, improve digestion, increase vitality, and reestablish the physiological balance that has been disturbed by nine months of pregnancy, labor, and delivery.
> - A daily routine that includes plenty of rest to protect the mother and focus her attention on properly nourishing herself and her baby during these first six weeks.
> - Vedic principles of baby care, including abhyanga, breast-feeding, and weaning.

There are special times in a woman's life when nature opens a narrow window, an opportunity for total rejuvenation of the physiology. These include the time just following the first menstrual period, the time of menopause, and the first six weeks after giving birth. This opportunity comes and goes regardless of whether one is aware of it or not. During these times, the woman's physiology is so delicate and sensitive that it is open and receptive to all influences. The simple but comprehensive regimen of the Mother and Baby program offers an opportunity for the woman's body to receive a total rejuvenation, thus alleviating the root causes of future disorders such as insomnia, indigestion, depression, etc. The body gets back into balance on the level of the doshas and all other aspects of the mind and body.

Advice from an Obstetrician

Rebecca Douglas, M.D., F.A.C.O.G., a board certified obstetrician with her own practice in Washington, D.C., herself followed the Mother and Baby program after the births of her two children, now ages five and eight. She also recommends it to her patients.

"I think the modern medical system does very little to support a woman during postpartum," she says. *"The obstetric prenatal care is excellent, but basically once the delivery has happened and she spends her astoundingly short one or two days in the hospital, we say, 'I'll see you in six weeks.' I just think that's cruel. It's a time when a woman has a lot of questions, a lot of insecurities, and is physically depleted—and there's not a conventional treatment for that woman.*

"To be an ideal citizen and an ideal mother we first have to be enlightened and rested in ourselves. This is for the baby's well-being, it's not an indulgence.

"I recommend the Mother and Baby program as an opportunity for the mother to be mothered, for the mother to get a much-needed rest and rejuvenation so that she has energy to give to the rest of the family.

"Particularly in the postpartum period, her first act of being a mother—and all subsequent acts—will be to give. And as mothers we can only give from what we have. And if what we have is exhaustion, then we'll have less of a basis from which to give. If, on the other hand, we have a methodology to rest and rejuvenate and give rest to ourselves, then we'll have that much more to give.

"I notice more enthusiasm, more vitality among my patients who follow the Mother and Baby program. A lot of the very immediate postpartum experience for any mother is that of euphoria. As time goes on and sleep deprivation mounts, by four weeks a lot of women's euphoria is pretty much suppressed and exhaustion takes over. So by the time I see them at six weeks postpartum, one of the most common questions I hear is, 'When is the baby going to sleep through the night?'

"For the women who go through the Mother and Baby program, how-

ever, that is not the common question I'm asked. Instead, I see much more of the "in-love" feeling that comes with being a new mother, the feeling of just being enthusiastic and infatuated with the new child. That tenderness and enthusiasm seems much more predominant and the fatigue seems to be much less."

Benefits of the Mother and Baby Program

Mothers who have enjoyed this program just can't stop talking about it. They cite benefits such as a complete revival of their normal energy levels, feeling blissful instead of depressed or overwhelmed, overcoming insomnia, receiving immediate relief from postpartum aches and pains, being able to breast-feed and bond with their babies more easily, and returning to their pre-pregnancy weight more rapidly. Even mothers who have had very difficult births are able to recover more quickly and completely with this program.

Madeleine, age 36, says, *"The first time around it was a much harder birth. I was in labor a long time, pushing a long time, and my body really got wiped out. I had terrible, all-the-time-pain for at least a year. I just felt awful all the time. With the first baby, the birth caused a very severe Vata or nervous system imbalance. My baby woke me up during the night for almost two years, so I couldn't sleep. He had terrible colic, too.*

"With my second son, who is now only six months old, I had the Mother and Baby program, which was wonderful. This baby is completely different. He's very quiet, he's been sleeping since the very beginning, and he has no colic.

"The first thing I noticed after the first treatment was a huge increase in energy.

"I also noticed that when I had a chance to rest, I slept much deeper. Now when I get a chance to close my eyes, my body is able to really settle down. Also, with this baby I've already lost all the weight and it's only been six months. With my first son it took two years.

"I felt it was intensely rejuvenating. I also experienced a soothing feeling at a very deep level. Not only physically—I felt soothed emotionally as well."

An Interview with a Mother and Baby Program Technician

Karen Oelberg lived in Vermont for five years and offered the Mother and Baby program to new mothers there. Most of these women had never heard of Maharishi Vedic Medicine or the Transcendental Meditation technique before meeting Karen.

Here are some comments from mothers she treated:

"The abhyanga was like Heaven on Earth."

"I felt as though I were floating."

"I feel like I'm being reborn."

"This is the best I've felt for nine months."

Karen says, *"I always tell new mothers that it's really for their child that they're having the Mother and Baby program. Because a mother's physiology is so intimately connected with her child's, if the mother has these nourishing treatments the baby benefits far more than anyone can imagine. The mothers experience this once they have their first treatment. Half of the women I treated liked it so much that they wanted to become Mother and Baby program technicians themselves.*

"I found that with the treatments, mothers really bounced back quickly. Some mothers looked really dragged out when I first saw them, because they had been running to the grocery store, cleaning the house, and cooking since the day after they came home from the hospital. Often I found that new mothers don't even realize that they're out of balance. They just start to feel worried or depressed. Their bodies won't let them take the rest, and the fatigue keeps piling up. Once they have the Mother and Baby program, their bodies start to relax and they can start sleeping. They start to take care of themselves, and take the rest that they need. Mothers go from feeling that their whole body is out of balance to feeling rested and transformed in just three or four days.

"I saw over and over again how much new mothers appreciate the program, how they felt healed by it, and how it helped them become better mothers. The herbalized abhyanga, the diet, and the herbs all work together syner-gistically. It's a really powerful thing, and there is nothing else like it out

there. Most mothers are used to just struggling through the first months with their babies. They're not used to being pampered like that."

Scientific Research on the Mother and Baby Program

A recent research study showed that the Mother and Baby program (including the Transcendental Meditation program) had a significant positive effect on mothers. The study, which was conducted at Maharishi University of Management in Fairfield, Iowa, provides qualitative data from interviews with thirty-one women in Fairfield who gave birth from February 1993 to December 1995. Eighteen women were practicing the Transcendental Meditation technique and participated in the Mother and Baby program, and thirteen women did not participate in either program. The report includes interviews conducted at six and twelve weeks postpartum, on family relationships; maternal, emotional, and bodily changes; maternal energy; sleep quality; and health.

The study concluded that overall health, confidence and happiness in being a new mother, family relationships, relationships with other children, bodily and emotional stability—all improved significantly in the group that followed the Mother and Baby program, compared to the control group that did not receive any treatment. (Please see Appendix B for a summary of the study.)

Another research study shows that Maharishi Rejuvenation therapy (a program for the general public, introduced in Chapter One, which includes abhyanga and heat treatments similar to those used in the Mother and Baby program) developed more mental and physical balance. Subjects were found to improve in feelings of life satisfaction, mood, sociability, openness, and extroversion. They reported less stress and strain, irritability, and health worries. These are similar to results reported by new mothers who follow the Mother and Baby program. (See chart on p. 17.)

Also, if the mother is practicing the Transcendental Meditation program, she has an opportunity to recover much more quickly from childbirth. People who practice the TM technique recover from stressful experiences more quickly. They experience less depression, anxiety, emotional numbness and insomnia after stressful experiences.[50,51]

The Father's Role during Postpartum

The postpartum period can also be challenging for men. Fathers go through a period of adjustment after the new baby is born. One study found that new fathers suffered from more fatigue, irritability, headaches, difficulty concentrating, insomnia, nervousness, and restlessness when compared with other men.[52] So your husband also needs to keep himself as healthy as possible, ideally by practicing the Transcendental Meditation technique, going to bed early, and eating nutritious meals.

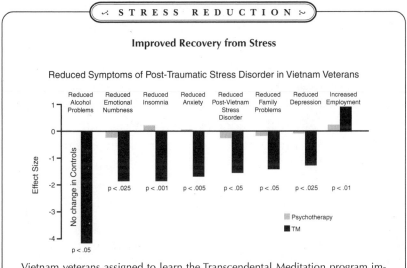

STRESS REDUCTION

Improved Recovery from Stress

Reduced Symptoms of Post-Traumatic Stress Disorder in Vietnam Veterans

Vietnam veterans assigned to learn the Transcendental Meditation program improved significantly on eight psychological and social measures, including reduced family problems and reduced depression, compared to other Vietnam veterans participating in psychotherapy. The first group also showed a more rapid physiological recovery from stressful stimuli.

Reference: J.S. Brooks and T. Scarano, "Transcendental Meditation in the Treatment of Post-Vietnam Adjustment," *Journal of Counseling and Development*, 64 (1986), pp. 212-215.

The father's support is absolutely essential at this time, and if possible, he should take at least a week's paternity leave to help you and your baby get settled.

He can help in many ways, mostly by giving nurturing care and attention to you and the baby. His main focus, in fact, should be to help you rest, because you need to rest in order to care for your baby properly. You also need his love and support, need him to be with you and the baby, sharing the bonding process, helping with diapering and rocking the baby, etc.

It's ideal if the two of you can arrange in advance to have someone clean, cook, and do the laundry during the delicate first weeks after birth. Then your husband is free to support you and help with baby care. Or if this is not possible, he can share in doing the household chores. He also should make sure your home is kept warm, as the baby is still adjusting to the cooler temperature outside the womb. You, too, will probably need greater warmth and nourishment to recover from extreme exhaustion.

Both parents need to make sure that any older children are receiving enough affection and attention as they adjust to having a new baby brother or sister. Their father can also help make them feel special by giving the older children extra attention.

During the first two weeks after delivery, when coming in from the working world, it's better if the father can bathe and change clothes before being with you and the baby. If this is not possible, he should at least wash his hands. This will ensure that germs, pollens, dust, grime, or toxins will not be introduced into the environment, protecting you and the baby from unnecessary exposure.

Sexual relations are not recommended for six weeks after birth, until the tissues heal and recover. *Sushruta Samhita* recommends that immediately after giving birth the mother should forgo sexual intercourse and physical labor of any kind. She should not allow herself to be angry or anxious, or to strain mentally in any way.

In this chapter we have seen how the Mother and Baby program recognizes that the postpartum period is a special time in a woman's life when nature opens a narrow window, an opportunity for total rejuvenation for the physiology. In the next chapter, we will provide simple but comprehensive recommendations for taking advantage of this opportunity, thus alleviating the root causes of future disorders.

Summary

The *Maharishi Ayur-Veda* Mother and Baby program provides the missing link in modern obstetrics. With simple, natural procedures it gives the mother the loving care she needs to recover from the exertion of giving birth, so she can give her new baby the nourishing, tender love that she feels in her heart.

"The effectiveness of Maharishi's Vedic Approach to Health lies in its ability to utilize the total intelligence of Natural Law at the basis of the human physiology— to utilize that holistic value of Natural Law that structures the physiology, and integrates the functioning of all aspects of body and mind. As a result, thought and behavior are spontaneously more in harmony with Natural Law, which is the basis of good health."

—*Maharishi Mahesh Yogi*[53]

CHAPTER ELEVEN

Why New Mothers Sometimes Feel Depressed

Carrie was young, healthy, and looking forward to the birth of her first baby. She expected to be the perfect mother—nourishing, energetic, and most of all, happy. Nothing prepared her for what happened next.

"With my first child, I felt really, really rough after the baby was born," she says. *"And I didn't expect it to be as rough as it was. I felt depression, and I definitely had a lot of freedom issues come up. I thought, 'I'm going to be stuck with this baby, and I'm not going to be able to go out and have fun any more or work.' There were a lot of tears, and it was very emotional. It was not as comfortable as it could have been. It was a rough birth as well. I had no help or anything afterward. I had a C-section, and that makes it even tougher because you don't bounce back as fast. I felt incredibly fatigued."*

Fortunately for Carrie, who is now 44 and the mother of three, she was able to avoid postpartum depression after the birth of her second and third children, even though they were also born by Caesarean section. Before the birth of her second child, she learned about the Mother and Baby program, and followed the simple recommendations of her physician trained in Maharishi Vedic Medicine.

"With the second child I took the Maharishi Ayur-Veda herbs, did my own abhyanga [oil massage], followed the postpartum diet, and took herbs

recommended by my physician. And I had so much energy. Just the herbs alone—it was incredible. The contrast between the two postpartum periods was like day and night. Plus I had help in the house. A couple of friends came over to make meals—I had company. I think that is another thing the Mother and Baby program offers. It recommends that new mothers have the support of other women, whereas I was left alone after the first birth. Having female companionship made a huge, huge difference.

"The third birth was the nicest, the smoothest of all. My stepdaughter watched my new baby for me while a Mother and Baby program technician give me my massage, every day for two weeks. It was lovely. I noticed the Mother and Baby massage got rid of my anxiety. I'd wake up in the morning and I'd feel spacey and filled with anxiety. I'd think, 'OK, I'm going to this today, and this and this and this.'

"But after the massage I just wanted to take a nap. Some of the time I was able to fall asleep after the massage. I also could sleep deeply at night. What I realized is that after giving birth, my Vata dosha was completely out of balance. I was so tired and wound up that when the technician finished massaging me and the Vata was back in balance, then I was able to relax and release the deep fatigue from childbirth and surgery.

"Whereas before, with my first child, I couldn't relax so I couldn't rest. I'd be running around doing much more than I should. And the tiredness and anxiety kept building and building. With the abhyanga, I didn't feel so anxious so I was able to take the rest I needed. I felt blissful instead of depressed."

Let's examine why these simple, natural recommendations could have such a big effect on Carrie and the hundreds of other mothers who have followed the Mother and Baby program during the past ten years.

Research on Postpartum Depression

There is significant research on the postpartum period. What it shows is that 80 percent of all mothers in America experience "postpartum blues"—a mild depression accompanied by crying, mood swings, irritability, anxiety, and inability to think clearly in the first two to ten days postpartum.[54]

This points to a definite gap in postpartum care. For most women in America who have a normal, uncomplicated birth, their hospital stays will last only one or two days. While this suits many women who want to be in their own home with their baby, it is terrifying to others who suddenly have to care for the baby on their own.

In fact, the current system expects mothers suddenly to become independent at the time they feel most vulnerable due to extreme fatigue, sleep deprivation, and emotional dependence. While mothers are often the center of attention when they are pregnant, even pampered and honored, now they are suddenly expected to care for a newborn and run the household when they feel least able.

Following are some of the common concerns expressed by new mothers—especially first-time mothers—reported in recent research on postpartum care in America:[55]

- Fatigue and sleep deprivation
- Feeling unable to cope with responsibilities of household, family, work, social relationships, and baby care long after the six-week postpartum period
- Lack of emotional, mental, or physical support
- Physical pain from hemorrhoids, episiotomies, back strain
- Anxiety, tension, mood swings
- Problems with breast-feeding or bonding
- Feeling unprepared to care for their baby on their own
- Anxiety about weight gain during pregnancy.

The worst thing is that the depression and fatigue tend to plague women long after delivery. Research shows that the majority of women still reported concerns about fatigue and tension between four and eight weeks postpartum. Feelings of depression continued during the third postpartum week, with 65 percent still feeling depressed by the eighth week.[56] Other studies found that women at three months still experienced physical discomfort, fatigue, depression, nervousness, difficulty adjusting to the needs of their baby and other children, and anxiety about their ability to cope.[57]

While the "baby blues" are experienced by the majority of women in America, a small percentage (about 10 percent) of these mothers develop severe enough depression that they can't care for themselves or their children.[58] Researchers have not located a clear cause of postpartum depression, and psychoanalysis seems to have little effect in improving the condition. One researcher, J. Errante, linked postpartum depression to sleep deprivation.[59]

This seems to make the most sense, because when someone is sleep deprived, they begin to show signs of stress. Sleep-deprived people become depressed, apathetic, and irritable, show increased sensitivity to pain and discomfort, display poor judgment, and even become aggressive.

Interestingly enough, Errante found that sedatives created a distorted sleep pattern that interferes with REM (Rapid Eye Movement) sleep. That's why some experts think that sleep medication actually makes insomniacs feel worse.

Instead, Errante suggested that sleep be promoted with warm milk, deep breathing, warm baths, massage, and a quiet environment. This is exactly what Maharishi Vedic Medicine recommends.

Causes of Postpartum Depression from the Perspective of Maharishi Vedic Medicine

The traditional Vedic view is that the postpartum period, when the mother's body is undergoing serious rebuilding, lasts for about six weeks after delivery.

During pregnancy, the embryo absorbs a large percentage of the mother's nutritional intake, leaving her own body depleted of nutrients. While all three doshas are involved in delivery, the tremendous effort of giving birth puts a great challenge on Vata dosha. You'll remember from previous chapters that Vata dosha governs all movement in the body. Specifically Apana Vata, which is the downward force responsible for moving the baby down the birth canal, is disturbed during the extreme exertion of giving birth, and often, as a result, the other aspects of Vata are disturbed, too.

After delivery, there is also a loss of blood when the placenta separates from the uterus and is discarded by the body. The volume of fluid and blood lost during the birth disturbs Vata, Pitta, and Kapha. The entire process leaves every cell depleted, and the woman feeling weak and undernourished.

Also, Vata gets thrown out of balance by irregular sleeping, waking, and eating patterns (which are inevitable when a new baby arrives). Other related factors are overwhelming physical and emotional demands, and sleep deprivation. So postpartum depression, you could say, is caused primarily by imbalance of Vata.

You'll remember from Chapter Three that when Vata goes out of balance, some of the symptoms include fatigue, anxiety, worry, insomnia, and constipation.

It's interesting that these are the exact symptoms that new mothers experience. The extreme exhaustion and fatigue, if not properly treated, can escalate into postpartum blues and even depression.

That's why Maharishi Vedic Medicine prescribes Vata-pacifying measures to bring the mother's body back into balance. Ways to keep Vata in balance include getting lots of rest, drinking plenty of warm liquids, eating three warm meals a day, staying in a calm, quiet environment, dressing warmly, and avoiding stimulating foods and situations. Specific measures are recommended for new mothers: gentle oil massage, warm baths, herbs, and a special diet to build up her depleted body and alleviate Vata dosha. These will help to bring her back to her normal level of health and energy.

Also, people who practice the Transcendental Meditation program experience less depression, because they are able to gain deep rest (both during meditation and at night) and release stress. Many of my patients report that the deep rest experienced during the TM technique helps them recover more quickly from the extreme fatigue after giving birth, and replaces it with more bliss and balance.

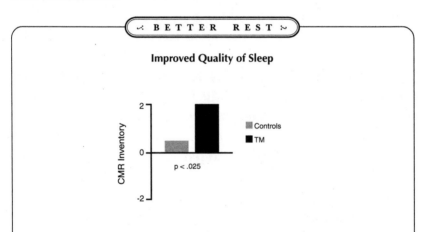

⪡ BETTER REST ⪢

Improved Quality of Sleep

In two companies that introduced managers and employees to the Transcendental Meditation program, those who practiced it regularly over a three-month period reported significantly greater reductions in health problems such as headaches and backaches, and improvements in quality of sleep. This is a natural consequence of reduced stress, and supports similar findings in other studies.

References: 1. C.N. Alexander, G. Swanson, M. Rainforth, T. Carlisle, and C. Todd, "The Transcendental Meditation Program and Business: A Prospective Study," paper presented at the 101st Annual Session of the Iowa Academy of Sciences, April 1989, Storm Lake, Iowa.
2. J. Fuson, "The Effect of the Transcendental Meditation Program on Sleeping and Dreaming Patterns," *Scientific Research on the Transcendental Meditation and TM-Sidhi Program: Collected Papers*, vol. 2 (Netherlands: MVU Press, 1989), pp. 880-896.
3. T. Haratani and T. Henmi, "Effects of Transcendental Meditation (TM) on the Health Behavior of Industrial Workers," *Japanese Journal of Public Health*, vol. 37, no. 10 (1990), p. 729.

You could think of the mother as being as delicate as a flower. She needs only rest, warmth, and serenity. Because the mother is in such a delicate condition after giving birth, Vedic texts recommend that she be nourished and protected. In fact she needs to be treated as protectively as the newborn child. This is especially true because the occurrence of any disease in a woman shortly after delivery can lead to disastrous consequences.

I have found over and over in my family practice that women will say, "I know this sounds silly, but I used to be very healthy until I had my baby. Ever since then I have had one health problem after another."

The Maharishi Vedic Approach to Health has an explanation for this. After giving birth, care must be taken to correct imbalances and strengthen the physiology. If that is not done, these imbalances can easily become aggravated, and thus a woman can become prone to one health problem after another. That is why the emphasis is on prevention. During this time, the mother should be very careful with her diet and daily routine, and should take the Maharishi Ayur-Veda herbs that have been recommended, so that she can return to her normal level of energy as soon as possible.

There is some interesting research on the effects of massage, heat treatments, herbs, and other therapies of the Maharishi Vedic Approach to Health. One study tested sixty-two subjects before and after they participated in Maharishi Rejuvenation therapy for one week, compared to seventy-one controls who received only intellectual knowledge during the same time period. Using the Profile of Mood States, it was found that those receiving Maharishi Rejuvenation therapy showed a significant increase in vigor and a significant decline in unhealthy emotional states such as anxiety, depression, fatigue, and confusion. This indicates that Maharishi Rejuvenation therapy improves the mind and emotions simultaneously.

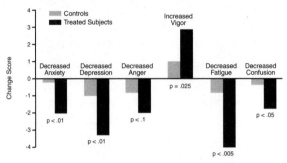

⤳ IMPROVED STABILITY AND VITALITY ⤳

Improved Health through *Maharishi Rejuvenation* **Therapy**

Two studies examined a combined total of 202 experimental subjects who had undergone 1-2 weeks of Maharishi Rejuvenation therapy, and compared them to a combined total of 131 controls who participated only in informational classes. The experimental subjects showed significant declines in unhealthy emotional states, improvements in appetite and digestive patterns, and increases in vigor, rejuvenation, and youthfulness.

Reference: R.H. Schneider, K.L. Cavanaugh, H.S. Kasture, S. Rothenberg, R. Averbach, D. Robinson, and R.K. Wallace, "Health Promotion With a Traditional System of Natural Health Care: Maharishi Ayur-Veda," *Journal of Social Behavior and Personality*, vol. 5, no. 3 (1990), pp. 1-27.

Turning the Postpartum Blues into Postpartum Bliss

It is interesting that women who follow these simple recommendations can enjoy the opposite of postpartum depression. Some people even report that they feel *better* and *healthier* since having their baby, once they followed the Mother and Baby program.

Sharon Thomas, former director of the Mother and Baby program says, *"I was extremely impressed because I never saw an instance of postpartum blues or depression in all of the years I worked with this program, and postpartum blues is normally quite common. Mothers looked healthier, just more supported, more rested. Their ongoing good health seemed to continue for years later. I have heard mothers say to me that they wanted to become pregnant so they could support and balance their systems through the Mother and Baby program. I literally heard this many, many times throughout the years. They wanted that opportunity to create new life and to reestablish balance in their own bodies. It's a window of opportunity that doesn't exist at other times."*

Postpartum Care in Other Cultures

We get so used to our own way of doing things that it's sometimes hard to believe that others would consider our ways strange. Although the postpartum period is not given a lot of attention in modern obstetrics, many traditional cultures view it as an extremely critical time in a woman's life, and give her as much support during that time as during pregnancy.

In Haiti, for instance, the crucial period of childbearing is after the baby is born. It is felt that the new mother needs special care to keep her body rested and warm after birth. She rests in bed for three days and in the subsequent weeks eats special warming foods, dresses warmly, takes various kinds of baths, and drinks warm herbal teas.

It's interesting that in several Eastern cultures—India, China, Laos, and Malaysia—these two themes, staying warm and resting after birth, are also emphasized. In these cultures, women are encouraged to rest for thirty to forty days, just taking care of themselves and their new babies while others prepare the food and take care of household duties. Massage is also mentioned in Malaysian and Indian postpartum studies. The Chinese believe that if a mother rests and remains at home, taking proper care of herself for a month after delivery, she will prevent future diseases related to the imbalances created during the pregnancy and delivery. The attention on keeping the mother warm and allowing her to rest deeply corresponds to the recommendation from the Mother and Baby program to balance Vata—which is active, cold, and dry—during this period.

I know, from growing up in India, that traditionally a few weeks before the child is due, the mother and her children go to her parents' home where she is really nurtured and taken care of in all respects—not only by her parents but by her siblings, extended family members, and friends. The mother is pampered, gets adequate rest and love, and prepares for the delivery. Her husband comes for the delivery. Since the period following birth is taken as a time of rest for the mother, the husband just visits and then returns home to work.

After the delivery in a hospital, the woman stays at the parents' home for the next four to six weeks postpartum to recuperate. The baby needs an extraordinary amount of care at that time—and there is lots of help around. The mother stays with her family until she has regained strength and can take care of the baby and the responsibilities of running the household. In India, even after the delivery, women in the family cook special foods for the new mother. In every household the grandmothers know the foods that reduce Vata dosha and balance the mother after giving birth.

Even with the advent of women working and the extended family nucleus being shattered in the major cities of India, there still is a lot of support from the community and relatives for the pregnant and postpartum mother. If the mother works, the parents or in-laws come to her house instead of her visiting them. Usually people in the community or the neighborhood will come and offer help, cook meals, take care of the children and provide whatever help they can. It seems to be a cross-cultural tradition that pregnant and postpartum females need to be nurtured and helped. When she first becomes pregnant, the mother starts planning how to get help after the baby is born.

The postpartum period is a critical time of bonding not only for the mother and baby, but also for the siblings. In India this is a period when the grandparents and aunts and uncles spend more time with the other children, saying again and again that "the new baby is a very important member of the family, you need to love him and take care of him." Every day this message keeps getting repeated to the older siblings. And the parents and in-laws constantly remind the husband that his wife needs more rest, more care. There is always a concerted effort on the part of the whole family to protect the mother and the child. Having the extended family there at the time of birth creates an extra bonding, extra strength and love for the whole family.

In my own case, long before my training in Maharishi Vedic Medicine, my mother-in-law was able to come to America in time for the delivery and was a source of great help, because I had to go back to work within two to three weeks. This was much too early. My body didn't feel rested or recovered yet, but with the help of my mother-in-law, I was able to manage.

Later, when I had my twin daughters, both my parents came to help. It was an extraordinarily challenging time for me because I had a complicated pregnancy and delivery, and it took me several weeks to recuperate. I received so much love and support from my parents—and truly I could not have managed the twins without their help, even though we had a live-in babysitter at that time. Having a two-year-old and the twin babies was a tremendous amount of work, and I was not able to do much of anything around the house because I was so extremely fatigued. My husband was a surgical resident at the time, which meant that he had very little time free to spend at home. My parents took responsibility for the household duties, and took care of the children with the help of the babysitter. That relieved much of the strain, and I could focus on my own recovery.

I am convinced that the reason there is very little postpartum depression in India is because at the birth of a baby all the members of the family support the mother, and young and old rejoice and celebrate. In the Vedic tradition, the birth of a baby is perceived as a cosmic event, and every baby is thought to be divine. When a child is born, the family affectionately addresses the baby as "Little Rama" or "Little Sita," or other names of the divine. It is felt that the baby brings good fortune, happiness, and evolution for the entire family. Based on that simple notion there is un-bounded joy—causing everyone to treat the child as precious. This creates continued waves of happiness for the mother. Every-one dotes on the new baby and praises him or her.

I also believe that in America, the high rate of postpartum blues or depression is caused by lack of rest, not knowing how to take care of the baby, and not receiving enough help and sup-port. Just because she is a woman doesn't mean that she will really understand what it means to have a baby. Most women don't fully understand this until they give birth. Even though it is a happy oc-casion, it is also a sudden shock when the baby arrives, because it is a totally new and different reality, which can be overwhelming. If the new mother has to deal with all these new responsibilities herself, it's too much to expect. If the husband and others help, then there is so much joy all around.

But how can all of this be arranged? The next chapter explains how.

Summary

The postpartum period doesn't have to be a time of fatigue, depression, and discomfort. If the mother is properly cared for, she can actually attain a state of health and energy beyond what she experienced before pregnancy.

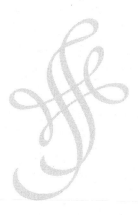

"The purpose of the Maharishi Vedic Approach to Health is to restore and maintain balance. Balance is the natural state of life, because the basic characteristic of the fundamental element of life, pure consciousness, is complete balance."
—Maharishi Mahesh Yogi

CHAPTER TWELVE

The "Rest, Rest, Rest" Routine for Postpartum

Now that you understand the reasons for postpartum fatigue and depression, you can organize your own postpartum recovery period carefully to avoid getting too tired. Above all, new mothers need rest. You can nap when your baby naps; start your evening routine early so you can fall asleep in the early evening, particularly if you'll have to be getting up in the night; and practice the Transcendental Meditation program morning and evening. You may think that you will never have time to meditate with a new baby—but it's more important now than ever before. You can meditate while your baby is napping. And you'll welcome the deep rest!

So important is this time for resting that Vedic texts recommend that both mother and baby stay mostly indoors for the first few weeks. (It is fine to walk in your yard if the weather is warm and the surroundings are fairly settled.) This is to protect your child from crowds and noise. Your new baby needs to make a transition from the womb, and it's best to take into account his or her delicate, sensitive nervous system.

This quiet routine gives the mother and child a chance to adjust to each other and enjoy each other without so much external stimulation and distraction. Mothers who follow this recommendation find that it gives them much more time to rest and recuperate.

Another reason to stay at home is that you can control the influences you subject your new baby to. Just as you avoided negativity while your baby was in the womb because it could affect his or her health, you'll want to create a protective, nourishing, loving environment now. This is such a tender time, when your every impulse is riding on a tender wave of love for your child. You want to avoid harsh emotions such as anger, worry, or fear—anything that might cast a shadow on your delicate feelings. Remember that one of the characteristics of Vata dosha is worry, so if you're worried the best thing is to calm Vata by resting. Staying at home can help you avoid getting too wrapped up in running errands and "getting things done" when you should be resting or playing with your newborn.

Of course, everyone is going to want to see the new baby. While this is a joyous time for celebration, it's also a time when long conversations can wear you out. You'll feel better if you don't try to keep up socially for these first few weeks. And remember that it's your job to keep a quiet, soft atmosphere so your baby can feel relaxed and comfortable.

In these first precious weeks, you may want to limit visitors to your immediate family and close friends—and just for a few hours a week in the afternoon, when your baby is likely to be napping. Make sure that visitors don't expect you to entertain them with meals or drinks. After all, you have the rest of your life to entertain your family and close friends—but only this one precious time to help your body recover and to create a beautiful relationship with your new baby.

Organizing for Help

One of the keys to a restful and joyful postpartum is to arrange for your household duties to be taken care of, as well as the main meal. This may sound harder than it actually is to do. If you have the means, you can hire someone to do the cleaning, laundry, cooking, and errands for a few weeks. Or if you have close friends or a family member (such as parents or a sister or aunt) living nearby, that would be ideal, because they would enjoy being near the baby and would do their tasks with love.

Your husband can also help, but remember that if he is working during the day and up during the night with the baby, he will need time to recuperate, too. And he needs time to enjoy his new child. Most of all, he needs to feel rested enough to give you the emotional support and care you need in order to be the best mother possible.

So it's better if someone else helps keep the household running just for these few weeks. You'll feel much better about yourself if your house is clean and orderly. Rather than struggling to keep up, it's better to *plan ahead* so you can focus on your real job during the six-week postpartum period—taking care of yourself and your baby.

In some areas, women form support groups to help each other with meals after the baby is born. In Fairfield, Iowa, where the first Maharishi Ayur-Veda Health Center was established in 1984, and where hundreds of women have benefited from the Mother and Baby program, it has become commonplace for the friends of the new mother to cook meals for her and her family for the first six weeks after the birth. If enough people help, each person only has to cook one or two meals over that period. All the support and love from friends and neighbors also helps nourish the new mother.

One mother from Fairfield says, *"I've been in communication with a pen-pal group on the Internet for moms throughout the country who want to share ideas for raising their kids. Almost every single mom was writing about the isolation of the postpartum period. I thought, 'What isolation?' Here in Fairfield I had six weeks with a gentle, kind technician giving me a massage and the neighbors cooking for me. When I wrote about my experience with the Mother and Baby program, these other moth-*

ers responded, 'Excuse me?' They wanted me to write articles for a newsletter about my experience. They could not believe that this was happening in this country.

"The Mother and Baby program gives you time for yourself, which is unusual for a new mother. You learn that you deserve to have someone come and help you with the housework during this exciting but fatiguing time. This program puts the mother in the supreme position—it holds motherhood very high. And that only helps you be a better, more loving mom."

Abhyanga for the New Mother

Abhyanga, the special oil massage described in Chapter Seven, is healthy for everyone, but especially for a mother who has just delivered her baby. Abhyanga is essential for the first twelve days in particular, because the massage increases circulation, bringing more oxygen and nutritive blood to every cell. This quickly aids in balancing the whole system, developing immunity, and strengthening the new mother.

Massage in general has been found by researchers to increase comfort and relaxation, improve circulation and drainage of lymph glands, prevent skin breakdown, condition the skin and muscles, and produce a state of well-being in mind, body and emotions. Massage reduces blood pressure and heart-rate,[60] and increases the skin temperature. It elevates mood and reduces distress from pain or physical symptoms.[61] Also, the sesame oil used in the Mother and Baby program is infused with calming herbs to soothe the new mother. The women who have been lucky enough to have this program have enjoyed huge shifts in their level of comfort soon after their first massage.

Andie, a new mother at 31, described her experience with the abbhyanga: *"After the birth of my daughter, I felt as though I had just been run over by a truck. But after just one abhyanga, all the fatigue was taken away. All the stress of delivery—that thick layer of fatigue—was gone, peeled away like the layers of an onion."*

Joan, who was 32 when her son was born, remembers that right after giving birth she was so tired that she thought she wouldn't have the abhyanga her husband had arranged for her. *"But the Mother and Baby program technician said 'No, it will be good for you—especially because you are tired.' And that very first day I felt completely rejuvenated. I felt life flooding back into my cells again. It was so nourishing and so rewarding for my body. I had a lot more energy and I felt really good."*

Valerie, age 41 when her baby was born, says, *"I felt that I could not have survived without the Mother and Baby program, especially since my baby had colic and I didn't get much sleep. The daily abhyangas really helped strengthen me, keeping me centered, giving me enough energy and clarity of mind to help me through. It was stabilizing, nurturing, comforting, balancing. On the days that I didn't have treatments I felt much more fatigue. The treatments made me feel that I could continue gracefully in my role as mother instead of just barely struggling through."*

Exercise

Basically, you'll just want to rest as much as possible and let your body tissues rebuild themselves during the first six weeks after delivery. If there has been any tearing during the birth, you will need to be especially careful about resuming your normal activities. If you have had a C-section, you will probably feel sore longer and will need even more time to heal.

After six weeks, if your physician agrees, you can start mild stretching exercises such as Yoga asanas (described in Chapter Seven). You'll want to build up gradually, giving your muscles a chance to recover. Walking in the fresh air is an excellent moderate exercise, which you can do even before six weeks has passed if you feel strong.

General Principles for Mothers
During the First Six Weeks Postpartum*

- Rest when the baby rests.
- Practice the Transcendental Meditation program twice daily.
- Give yourself a daily abhyanga, or better still, have a Mother and Baby program technician come to your home and give you one.
- After the abhyanga, nap for 20–30 minutes, setting hot water bottles on your lower back and abdomen. Then take a hot tub bath.
- Eat light, warm, liquid, easily digestible foods.
- Avoid worry and anger.
- Keep your activity settled and quiet.
- Try to limit visiting hours so you don't get too tired out.
- Stay at home as much as possible. Avoid going in crowded areas for at least three weeks. Avoid wind, cold, harsh lights, and dust.
- Try to arrange for someone to take care of the cooking, cleaning, and laundry for these first weeks, so you can rest and focus on nourishing your baby.
- Keep yourself and your baby warm. Wear slippers and sweaters inside your home.
- Start your evening routine early; then if your baby wakes up to nurse, at least you have a few hours of sleep before midnight.

---

*These guidelines are especially important during the first twelve days after birth, although it's ideal to continue them for six weeks postpartum.

Summary

By organizing your daily schedule so you can rest, practice the Transcendental Meditation technique, and have a daily abhyanga during the postpartum period, you can dramatically facilitate your recovery. By focusing on rest you can make optimum use of your ability to heal and recover most quickly.

"Milk is the best of all nutritive substances. Through its kindred or similar properties, it augments the quality of ojas in the body."   —*Sushruta Samhita*[62]

"Cold or unboiled milk is extremely heavy, and serves to increase the slimy secretions of the organs, whereas by boiling it is freed from those injurious traits."
                    —*Sushruta Samhita*[63]

CHAPTER THIRTEEN

Digestion, Food, and Herbs During Postpartum

Your diet becomes even more important if you are breast-feeding, because what you eat will affect your child's mental and physical health. According to Maharishi Vedic Medicine, different physical and mental factors directly affect the milk of the mother—its quantity of production as well as its quality. If for some reason your digestive power is not working properly, it could affect the metabolism of your child, causing minor and major illnesses ranging from colic to fever.

Also, it's important to eat the right foods, not only to restore balance, but because your digestive power is particularly weak at this time. Maharishi Vedic Medicine provides a diet that meets both of your needs simultaneously—the need to eat foods that will nourish your new baby through your milk, and the need to eat foods that will restore your weak digestion.

Your Digestion after Childbirth

After giving birth, you will probably find that your digestion is very delicate and weak. This is because the exhausting labor actually extinguishes the digestive fire.

Perhaps you remember from Chapter Six that this digestive power is called *agni*, which you could think of as being like a fire. During the birth process all of the energy normally used for digestion goes into pushing the baby out of the birth canal. Thus the fire of digestion gets nearly extinguished. So agni needs to be rekindled during the six-week postpartum period.

You can build your digestion not only by eating the right foods, but also by following the guidelines listed in Chapter Six. These include eating at the same time every day, eating your main meal at noon, eating in a settled and quiet atmosphere, and sitting down while you eat. All of these simple, natural recommendations will help get your digestion back to normal.

Benefits of the Postpartum Diet

Just as in pregnancy, there are specific doshas that need to be balanced during postpartum, so Maharishi Vedic Medicine outlines the specific foods that will meet a woman's specific needs and bring her body back into balance. The diet includes foods to strengthen your digestion and create healthy breast milk. You'll want to consult your physician/practitioner to receive a complete list of these special foods.

You may be thinking that you don't want to be on a diet while you are recovering from labor and using up extra calories. But it's not a "diet" in the sense of "feeling deprived." The foods recommended for postpartum by Maharishi Vedic Medicine are extremely satisfying, and most women find that they actually crave these exact flavors.

The best thing about this diet is that it is light and easy to digest, and at the same time nourishing and nutritious. That's why women who follow this diet tend to have an easier time returning to their prepregnancy weight while still eating all the nutrients and calories needed for breast-feeding. A new mother can gain a lot of nourishment without feeling overloaded with heavy food.

Also, these foods are simple to prepare. Best of all, you can eat as much as you want!

Cathy, a mother for the first time at age 39, says, *"For some reason these foods and seasonings really hit the spot. They were so light and easy to digest, yet they were so, so satisfying. I felt that the food was going straight to my cells, nourishing me and giving me energy to recover, breast-feed, and take care of my baby all at once."*

Many breast-feeding mothers notice that when they follow this diet, their babies do not have colic. This is because if the mother eats foods that are easy to digest and do not cause gas, her breast milk will cause less gas in her baby. Maharishi Vedic Medicine points out that there seems to be a direct correlation between the baby's digestion and the mother's diet and digestive strength.

"Diet made a big difference," says Karen, a 33-year-old mother of two. *"I followed the recommended postpartum diet to avoid constipation for myself and colic for the baby. If I went off the diet—for instance, if I ate anything with kale or cabbage or strong spices—the baby would get very cranky. This was true for both my children. If I strayed, the baby would fuss."*

Another mother, age 47, says, *"With my first child, I didn't know about the Mother and Baby program, so I didn't know that eating certain things would cause gas in my baby. I certainly learned fast. I remember one night waking up in bed to nurse and saying to my husband, 'I smell strawberries.' I had strawberry milk because I had just eaten strawberries that day. I realized then that you synthesize what you eat. My baby had terrible colic, and it was hard to isolate those things that made him cry. With the Mother and Baby program, you learn which vegetables and other foods make problems, and consequently my next two children didn't have a problem with colic."*

Foods to Include during Postpartum: In general, the postpartum diet includes foods that are cooked, soupy, fresh, organic if possible, and easy to digest. Delicious, warm, lovingly prepared foods that smell and look appetizing help stimulate the appetite.

Usually, it's recommended to eat a diet that includes more sweet tastes. Remember that "sweet" does not mean large amounts of sugar. Rather it means including more rice, milk, ghee, and easily digestible wheat products such as cream of wheat.

Cooked vegetables that are especially healthy during this time are beets, carrots, zucchini, sweet potato or yams, spinach, summer and winter squash, peeled tender eggplant, and asparagus. Cracked wheat cereal (bulgur wheat), cous cous, cream of wheat, raw sugar or dried cane juice (available in Indian groceries as *jaggary*), watery split-mung dahl, khichari (cooked rice and dahl together), and cooked sweet fruits are also good postpartum foods. You'll also want to prepare mung dahl and rice with more water than before. This makes them easier to digest.

For snacks, a few blanched almonds and some raisins, dates, and flaked coconut are nourishing and easy to digest. And they help to promote ojas (described in Chapter Six), create healthy breast milk, and rebuild the shukra (reproductive tissue).

Admittedly the postpartum diet is plainer than the average American diet, but it does include tasty, mild flavorings and spices that promote digestion and have calming effects. Spices such as fenugreek, fennel, saffron, cinnamon, coriander, cardamom, cumin, ginger, salt, clove, and small amounts of black pepper help improve digestion and at the same time make the food more enjoyable. Vata Churna is a prepared mixture of spices that is also an excellent flavoring for postpartum, as it includes all six tastes and is designed to balance Vata dosha.*

Foods to Avoid during Postpartum: In the past, you may have been in the habit of drinking cold liquids, but during postpartum you'll especially want to stay away from cold drinks and cold

---

*See Appendix C to order.

foods, because they increase Vata dosha and impair digestion, which is already sluggish during this time. You'll also want to stay away from raw, cold foods, and leftovers, as these are hard to digest and create *ama*, the sticky waste-product of undigested food that is the cause of many disorders.

As in pregnancy, sour and pungent tastes should also be avoided during postpartum. Sour foods include fermented or acidic foods, such as vinegar, yogurt, lemon, pickles, or aged cheese. Examples of pungent or hot, highly spicy foods include chili powder, garlic, and onions, and aromatics such as mint.

Meat is not recommended for the first twelve days, even if you are not a vegetarian. This is because meat is very difficult to digest. A vegetarian diet is ideal at this time. If you crave meat, try having chicken, turkey, or fish in soup form. Also avoid alcohol, coffee, carbonated drinks, and chocolate.

If you're breast-feeding, which Maharishi Vedic Medicine usually recommends, you'll especially want to avoid any gas-producing foods, because they can have the same effect on your baby. These include broccoli, cauliflower, cabbage, onions, garlic, brussels sprouts, potatoes, kale, green peas, green peppers, sprouts, and any raw vegetables (such as in salads).

Here's a sample menu:

Breakfast: Cream of rice or cream of wheat with milk, ghee and raw sugar or raw honey

Lunch: Rice
One cup of mung dahl
Sweet potato with ghee
Zucchini sauteed in ghee, fennel and coriander.
Apple crisp made with raw sugar

Dinner: Vegetable soup flavored with Vata churna
Cous cous

Remember When You are Breast-feeding . . .

When you are breast-feeding, it's important that you eat a bal-anced diet of whole grains, vegetables, fruit, and dairy products. It's essential to drink lots of water, and to drink lots of milk.

Milk is by far the most important food for a nursing mother, because it contributes directly to healthy breast milk. According to the Vedic texts, it gets converted directly to ojas. As discussed in Chapter Six, milk is more digestible if it is boiled first, and then drunk while still warm. This will help to make your own breast milk more nourishing. It's more digestible, too, if you add a little cardamom or ginger while it is boiling. Adding raw sugar or honey after it has cooled a bit will make a delicious and soothing drink. Drink organic milk if possible.

Even mothers who don't usually drink milk realize that they've actually been craving it when they drink it warm with ginger, ghee, and raw sugar.

Reminders for the Postpartum Breast-feeding Diet

- Be sure to follow the guidelines for a warm, nourishing, unctuous diet (described in Chapter Six).
- Eat fresh, organically grown, well-cooked, delicious, sat-isfying food.
- Eat it in pleasant company without rushing.
- Try to maintain regular mealtimes, as this aids digestion.
- Be relaxed and happy when eating.
- Be sure to drink lots of warm liquids, including purified water. (Breast-feeding mothers need up to two quarts of liquids a day.)
- Avoid foods that can cause gas.
- Eat more ghee and drink more milk than usual.

Losing Weight after Pregnancy

Of course you will be concerned about losing the excess weight that you gained during pregnancy. Usually, you will lose twelve to fifteen pounds with the birth of the baby (including the baby's weight, the placenta, and amniotic fluid).

If you are breast-feeding, it's not a good idea to go on a weight-loss diet, because you need the extra calories to feed your baby. A breast-feeding woman requires between 1,000 and 3,500 more calories per day than at other times in her life.[64] This is equivalent to the amounts needed when becoming an athlete or jogging ten miles.

The good news is that the postpartum diet recommended by Maharishi Vedic Medicine can provide all the nutrients and nourishment you need and help you lose weight at the same time. The reason that so many women find it difficult to lose weight after delivery is not because of the amount of food they are eating, but because their digestion is not strong.

As mentioned earlier, the digestive fire gets weakened in many women after delivery. Since digestion is somewhat delicate, if you don't put the proper foods in the system and take steps to balance the digestion, then the food you eat will not be digested properly and will build up ama in your body; and thus it will take longer to lose weight.

The key to losing weight is not to strain your body by going on a strict diet, but just to eat these simple, balanced, easy-to-digest foods that are nourishing. Also, you'll want to follow the recommendations in Chapter Six for strengthening digestion and resetting balance in this delicate area of life.

Hundreds of mothers have reported that they have returned to their pre-pregnancy weight much more quickly and effortlessly when they followed these simple principles. Once the body is balanced, then good health and normal weight naturally follow.

Toni, 31, says, *"What was also miraculous to me was that in just a few weeks after the baby was born I dropped all my pregnancy weight. I think a lot of that had to do with exercising regularly before pregnancy and following the Mother and Baby program once the baby was born. Everything just simply and easily went back into place."*

Herbal Compounds for Postpartum

Another aspect of the Mother and Baby program are herbal compounds (including an herbal tea) that are specifically formulated for postpartum women. These are designed to eliminate fatigue, enhance digestion, and promote healthy breast milk. You can order these and additional herbal supplements that your physician/practitioner may prescribe if you need them (see Appendix C). These strengthen the female tract and help restore balance to that area after giving birth.

Many women have enjoyed tremendous benefits from taking the herbal compounds and herbal tea to strengthen digestion and promote healthy breast milk. The herbs are natural and mild, and give an added boost to digestion right when a new mother needs it most. The herbal tea can also be given to the baby directly to help relieve gas.

Mona, mother of three, says, *"My children weren't exactly colicky, but I did give them the recommended herbal tea. For at least two of my kids that had good results. When they would cry, I would just give them the herbal tea, and they'd stop crying and kicking."*

Darlene, age 37, noticed that the herbal tea helped her own digestion. *"Following the births of both my children, I'd have cramps and pain in my stomach after I ate. The tea to aid digestion really seemed to help with that."*

Herbal and mineral compounds have been used since time immemorial, and are an important part of the Maharishi Vedic Approach to Health. Thousands of herbs are included in the *materia medica* of Maharishi Vedic Medicine.

Herbs have played an important role in other systems of medicine as well.

It is said that Hippocrates, the father of Western medicine, used twenty-nine of the three hundred known herbs of his time to cure all disease on the Isle of Cos. In addition to the ancient Greeks, the Romans, Egyptians, Chinese, and Native Americans were known for their herbal medicines.

Of the earth's estimated 600,000 plant species, only a small number are classified as herbs and used for healing. Herbs are the most refined products of the plant kingdom, and in combination contain all seventeen minerals and seventy trace minerals that the body needs to operate. Each herb has a frequency, or vibration, that matches the frequency or vibration of a certain part of the body. When the wave motion of a part of the body is out of sequence, that area of the body becomes out of balance. The correct herb can restore normal functioning. Each herb acts like a tuning fork, causing its target tissue to resonate at the proper frequency, thus reestablishing natural balance.

In Maharishi Vedic Medicine, herbs are used whole—either crushed, dried, cooked, or powdered in their entirety. This is because the whole plant creates a balanced effect in the body. This is opposite to the approach of Western medicine, which isolates and extracts the "active ingredient" from plants, creating a potent, imbalanced effect that can have strong negative side-effects on the body.

There's another important distinction between the Maharishi Ayur-Veda herbs and herbs you may purchase at a health food store. In Maharishi Vedic Medicine, herbs are usually combined in compounds that enhance their potency and create greater balance. These herbal formulas are carefully prepared according to the ancient Vedic texts, which contain specific directions for gaining the most value from the herbs. For instance, when heating herbs it's important not to let them get too hot so the nutritional value won't be destroyed. Some herbal compounds take days of constant attention to prepare properly.

The main purpose of Maharishi Ayur-Veda herbal compounds is to wake up the biological intelligence in the body, thus allowing the natural healing power of nature to bring the body back into balance. There are herbal compounds for the mind and emotions as well—for example, to enhance clear thinking or balance the emotions, both of which are crucial for new mothers.

Maharishi Amrit Kalash® Herbal Supplement: Maharishi Vedic Medicine's Most Powerful Herbal Compound

This two-part herbal supplement, Nectar herbal fruit concentrate and Ambrosia herbal tablets, is considered to be the cream of herbal preparations in Maharishi Vedic Medicine. Developed more than two thousand years ago, the two parts are complex formulas, containing between them more than fifty herbs and minerals. They are designed to root out the cause of disease by bringing the three doshas into equilibrium and to create balance throughout the whole mind and body.

These two are highly recommended for new mothers, because they help them to regain their strength and eliminate fatigue. And they have a powerful rejuvenating effect, boosting the immune system.

Here are some of the reported benefits of Maharishi Amrit Kalash herbal supplements:

- Slows premature aging
- Sharpens mental focus
- Combats stress
- Enhances natural beauty
- Increases alertness
- Reduces fatigue
- Elevates energy levels

- Improves creativity
- Restores inner calm
- Creates mental and physical balance
- Provides a sense of well-being

One of the reasons Maharishi Amrit Kalash food supplements can have such a profound effect on the whole system is that they help eliminate free radicals, one of the major underlying causes of disease. Free radicals are destructive molecules that cause cars to rust and the cells in the body to age and deteriorate. They attack the cell membrane, the DNA, and the mitochondria. Recent research is finding that as much as 70 percent of disease is caused by free radicals. Because free radicals become active when they combine with oxygen molecules, a combination of enzymes and nutrients called *antioxidants* are used to neutralize them. Antioxidant substances help to prevent heart disease, for example, by inhibiting oxidation of LDL (low-density lipoproteins, also commonly known as "the bad cholesterol") and other fats. Many people take antioxidant vitamins to fight the free radicals responsible for such oxidation. However, it takes huge quantities of Vitamin C or E to scavenge or neutralize free radicals, and even then only a limited range of free radicals is affected.

Now extensive research conducted at The Ohio State University College of Medicine and other leading institutions is showing that the Maharishi Amrit Kalash formulas are remarkably effective as antioxidants. Just to name a few of their antioxidant qualities, researchers have found that these formulas have 1,000 times more antioxidant power than known antioxidants Vitamin C or E.[65, 66] Also, you could think of the Maharishi Amrit Kalash formulas as "full-spectrum" antioxidants, which means that they are effective against hundreds of types of free radicals, not just a few select types. And while single-ingredient antioxidants work only either outside the cell or inside, Maharishi Amrit Kalash herbal supplements reach the entire cell.

After the Postpartum Period

You'll want to ease into your normal activities after the postpartum period. Some of the Mother and Baby program recommendations even can become regular parts of your normal daily routine, creating better health all the time.

Diet: You can follow the postpartum diet for a longer period if it is satisfying to you. Consult your physician/practitioner trained in Maharishi Vedic Medicine to see if it is the right long-term diet for your particular make-up and health needs. Usually, after six weeks, if you are not experiencing any digestive trouble or other symptoms of discomfort, your doctor will recommend that you return to the diet that you normally enjoy. Remember, though, that you are still breast-feeding your baby, so you will want to avoid junk food, empty calories, and processed foods that contain a lot of chemicals. Continue to favor organic fresh vegetables, fruits, whole grains, and dahls as much as possible.

Fluids: Remember to drink when you are thirsty. If you are continuing to breast-feed, be sure to maintain your one and one-half to two quarts of warm water per day.

Herbs: You can consult your physician/practitioner to see if you need any additional herbal supplements after completing the special postpartum herbs.

Daily Abhyanga: Because this enlivens and revitalizes your body, you'll want to continue your morning self-massage. It's recommended for your whole family to increase immunity and energy.

Seasonal **Maharishi Rejuvenation** *Therapy:* The purifying and eliminative treatments included in the Maharishi Rejuvenation program (panchakarma) are recommended for a few days every season. With these soothing abhyangas, steam baths, and gentle eliminative therapies, you can clear away the impurities and tox-ins that build up with each season before the new season begins.

Menstrual Cycle: Once your menstrual cycle starts again, Maharishi Vedic Medicine recommends that you follow a special diet each month during this time. You'll also want to get more rest to ensure a healthy cycle and to help your reproductive or-gans recover more quickly from pregnancy and childbirth. (Your physician/practitioner can advise you.) You'll want to avoid doing abhyanga at home during the first three days of your cycle each month because your body is already purifying. This is also true when you are sick.

Summary

After giving birth your digestion may be weaker than usual. By taking care to balance your body through special foods and herbal supplements, you can help your digestion work prop-erly—and create more energy for yourself and healthier breast milk for your baby.

PART III

New Baby Care

New Baby Care

During the past thirty years, a large quantity of research has come out on the relationship between mother and child, known as "bonding." A strong infant-maternal bond can have an enormous impact on the child, affecting his or her self-esteem, ability to form close relationships, and happiness.

A number of factors contribute to bonding, including the interaction with the mother in the first hours after birth, breast-feeding, and opportunities for loving touch. It's interesting that the *Maharishi Ayur-Veda* Mother and Baby program develops the exact conditions necessary for bonding, first by helping the mother stay rested and relaxed, and by recommending natural methods such as abhyanga (oil massage) to nourish her new baby.

In Chapter Fourteen, you'll learn about the infant's need for loving touch, and find out how to give your baby a daily abhyanga to promote strong immunity, relaxation, and emotional stability. Breast-feeding, weaning, and first foods are discussed in Chapter Fifteen. Chapter Sixteen discusses the recent research on bonding, and describes how the natural recommendations of the Mother and Baby program strengthen the mother-infant bond. Finally, in the last chapter of the book, you'll get a glimpse of the future your child can enjoy through Maharishi Vedic Medicine—a life free of stress, disease or unhappiness, a life of Heaven on Earth.

"The infant should be lifted gently and should not be scolded. He should not be awakened suddenly lest he might get frightened. He should not be snatched from others nor should he be thrown in the air lest Vata and other doshas get disturbed. He should not be made to sit very early lest he may suffer from kyphosis (curvature of the spine). He should always be consoled by hundreds of pleasing things so that he may not get annoyed.

"If the child is thus brought up according to his leanings, he develops a sharp intellect day by day, and becomes healthy and cheerful.

"The child should be protected from the wind, bright sun, lightning, trees, creepers, vacant houses, low-lying areas, and infections.

"The child should not be left in places which are dirty, open or uneven, nor should he be kept in a hot or windy place, nor in the rain, a dusty or smoky place or in water."   —*Sushruta Samhita*[67]

CHAPTER FOURTEEN

The Baby Massage

It is hard for an adult to appreciate how a newborn child might feel. Imagine if you just spent nine months in a dark, moist, protected, warm place. Probably it would take some time before you got used to bright lights and loud noises—or even to being left alone in a crib. Your newborn baby is in a very tender and delicate state in the first few weeks after birth, and you want to take every precaution to protect him.

Maharishi Vedic Medicine recommends that you keep your baby away from intense sensory stimuli during this time. This includes cold winds, drafts, bright sunlight, bright lighting, loud music, crowds, or even the smell of strong perfume. While it's healthy to take your baby outside to breathe fresh air if the weather permits, the newborn needs warmth, quiet, and no jarring stimuli, whether inside or outside. By protecting your baby from strong sensory input during the first six weeks, you can allow him to make the adjustment to life outside the womb at his own rate.

It may seem unusual to modern mothers to spend so much time quietly at home, away from work, shopping malls, or grocery stores. But it's only for a few weeks, and if you can possibly arrange it, it's well worth it. Staying home quietly with your baby also helps with the bonding process. This is a precious time to enjoy with your newborn—so you'll want to make the most of it.

The Maharishi Ayur-Veda Baby Massage (Abhyanga)

One of the most enjoyable things you can share with your baby is an abhyanga. The baby abhyanga is a gentle sequence of strokes designed to improve your baby's digestion, loosen muscular tension, and increase muscle strength.

The baby abhyanga is easy to do and has a profound effect on the baby. Babies thrive on it. And it gives you a chance to convey pure love to your child. For a baby, touch is a powerful means of communication.

It is evident to me as a physician, that babies treated with this massage enjoy a greater overall immunity. How does this happen? The skin is the largest organ in the body. The sense of touch is first experienced by the embryo at six weeks, before the eyes and ears develop. In the developing fetus the outermost of the three embryonic layers (the ectoderm) forms the central nervous sys-

---

Some Benefits of Baby Abhyanga

- Gently presses impurities out of the tissues into the channels of the body.
- Enhances circulatory system.
- Brings nourishing blood and oxygen to all cells of the body.
- Helps digestion—can help settle stomach pain or gas.
- Relaxes the baby and promotes deeper sleep.
- Tones the baby's muscles.
- Releases stress and tension caused by the baby's having been cramped in the fetal position in the womb.
- Facilitates and enhances communication, sharing, and bonding.
- Helps keep the baby settled and happy.
- The warm bath afterwards allows the channels to expand so the impurities can be released.

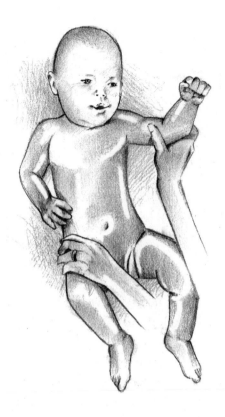

tem and then extends to cover the body in the form of skin, hair, nails, and teeth. Because the skin is something like an outer nervous system, it makes sense that gently massaging the skin could have such dramatic effects on the mind, emotions, and body.[68]

Guidelines for Baby Abhyanga

For complete instructions, it's best to receive direction from a physician trained in the Maharishi Vedic Approach to Health. Here are some basic points, including preparation, proper environment, the general approach to the massage, and materials:

After the umbilical cord falls off, you can start giving your child an abhyanga each morning, using warm sesame oil. The abhyanga normally takes five or ten minutes. You can also give your baby an abhyanga each evening before bed. This helps him or her relax and fall asleep more easily. Also, if there is any indigestion, this massage can help soothe and relieve gas. You don't need to give your baby a bath afterwards—just use less oil and gently stroke it on. Fathers often enjoy giving this evening massage after work. It's a great way for a new father to become comfortable handling and interacting with his newborn.

It's best to wait until half an hour after feedings to start the abhyanga. There are times when you'll want to skip the massage—such as when the baby has a cold or fever—but otherwise you can do it every day.

Preparation: You can set up an area in the bathroom for the baby abhyanga, with some towels on the floor to provide a soft, clean surface for the baby to lie on. Having a few extra towels handy to wipe your hands is a good idea.

Warm sesame oil is recommended for baby abhyanga, although in cases when the baby has sensitive skin or rashes, coconut oil or ghee is sometimes better. The oil should have been cured first (see Chapter Seven for directions). Plastic flip-top containers are excellent for holding the abhyanga oil. Warm the oil by placing the container in warm water. It should be pleasantly warm for the massage.

The room should also be quite warm. Babies are much more sensitive to cold than are adults. During the first month of life, even clothed babies need a minimum temperature of 75° in an area free from drafts. Usually, temperatures below that will be uncomfortable for the child. This is because the baby has less body mass to hold the heat, and will cool much more quickly than an adult. When you think about it, in nature mothers of mammals work hard at keeping their offspring warm.

Be sure your nails are pared and remove rings or any sharp jewelry that might scratch your baby.

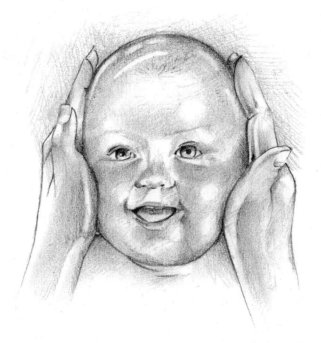

Giving the Abhyanga: Undress your baby and place her on the towel. As you do the baby abhyanga, speak gently and sweetly to your baby and let her know what you're doing, tell her how good she is and how much you love her. It's a precious time to share with your baby. Especially with newborns, use gentle and slow movements, as instructed by a physician/practitioner. As your baby grows older, she may roll over or sit up during the massage. This is to be expected and is no obstacle to giving an abhyanga. Remember, though, to support your baby's head and neck whenever you're the one changing her position. As with your own abhyanga, the general approach is to use a circular motion on the joints and long strokes on the limbs.

After the Abhyanga: Follow the abhyanga with a warm bath to wash off the excess oil. This will also open the channels of purification and allow impurities to be released from the tissues. Or you can give your child a sponge bath by soaking a towel in warm water and wiping the oil off gently.

Traditionally, Vedic texts recommend mild cleansers to remove the oil from the baby, such as chickpea flour (called gram flour in Indian grocery stores) and milk. However, the flour tends to clog drains, so be cautious. If you soak the chickpea flour in the milk while giving the abhyanga, it will absorb enough moisture to reduce its tendency to clog the drain. (Note: Regular flour won't work. If you can't find chickpea flour at a natural foods store or Asian grocery store, you can use a coffee/spice grinder to make a fine powder from red lentils or yellow split mung.) Warm water or warm milk is often enough by itself to remove the oil. In any case, it's better not to use soap on the newborn baby's delicate skin. Also, you don't need to wash her hair more than once a week. The oil actually protects the baby's scalp and head. It's a good idea to keep the head covered with a cotton cap, especially after massage, to protect from drafts.

Sesame Oil and the Skin

Sesame oil is recommended in the Vedic texts for abhyanga because it is nourishing, rejuvenating, and balancing to the skin and all the doshas. The oil provides a smooth, frictionless medium so the baby's tender skin never feels chafed.

Because the cell membrane is lipid soluble, fats such as sesame oil can penetrate it. As you massage your baby's skin, the fresh, pure sesame oil penetrates the pores of the skin and inner cell membranes, replacing the older lipid (fatty) molecules that make up the cell walls with new lipid molecules. This is one reason why sesame oil abhyanga is held to be so refreshing and rejuvenating—the older lipid molecules containing wastes get flushed away by fresh new oil molecules. You can see why it's important to use the highest grade of organic sesame oil.*

---

* See Appendix C to order.

Sesame oil also has a unique antibacterial quality, giving it a cleansing, purifying effect. Research studies on sesame oil have documented beneficial qualities that may explain why Vedic texts hold it in such high regard. One study found that sesame oil retards the growth of skin cancer;[69] another that it inhibits the growth of human colon cancer in vitro.[70]

Research on Baby Massage

During the past few years, there has been increasing public interest in baby massage. Hundreds of hospitals throughout the U.S. now offer infant massage for premature babies and teach parents how to massage their babies as part of their hospital stay for birth. Massage therapy schools and other organizations now teach infant massage. One national organization of infant massage therapists presently numbers 4000, and many therapists have set up institutes to teach massage to parents.

Tiffany Field, Ph.D., a leader in research on infant massage, comments, "We know now that infant massage helps growth and development. Babies who are massaged gain more weight, they sleep better, they are less irritable, they are more responsive, they have better interactions with their parents and they show superior mental and motor development."[71]

Dr. Field and her associates at the University of Miami and Duke University Medical Schools published a ground-breaking study in the journal *Pediatrics* in 1986. The researchers evaluated forty premature babies who were hospitalized for an average of twenty days. Half of the infants were exposed to body stroking and movement of their limbs for three fifteen-minute sessions per day over a period of ten days. Then they and a matched control group were given a series of tests.

As a result, the massaged babies averaged a 47 percent greater weight gain per day, even though they were fed the same amount of formula as the control group. They were also more active and alert, and showed more mature habituation, orientation, motor skills, and behavior than the control infants. And their hospital stays were six days shorter, yielding a cost saving of approximately $3000 per infant.[72]

Another study on premature babies was conducted by psychologist Ruth Rice, and involved teaching mothers to massage their preterm infants daily and rock them. At four months, the massaged babies were ahead in both neurological development and weight gain.[73] The natural sensory stimulation of massage speeded development of the brain and nervous system, improving mind-body integration.[74]

Very little research has been done on healthy infants, although massage therapists throughout the country report that infant massage facilitates the parent-infant bonding process; develops warm, positive relationships between mother and child; reduces stress; reduces colic; helps induce sleep; and provides parents with enjoyable experiences with their infants.

Some Mothers Talk About the Baby Abhyanga

In India where I grew up, abhyanga is practiced in virtually every home. Often the grandmother gives the baby the abhyanga, but if she doesn't live with the family, the mother does it. My own grandmother would set a stool in the shower, tie her sari up and place the baby on her legs. Then she'd swish the oil between her hands and massage her grandchild as he or she slid up and down her legs. She would also move the baby in mild stretching exercises, and put drops of oil in the ears and nose. Then the baby would sleep like a rock, being so deeply rested! One of my earliest memories is of my grandmother massaging me at age three months.

My family also used aroma therapy to soothe the mother and baby and help with sleep.

Once you start massaging your infants, you don't have to stop as the children grow older. My twin daughters are teenagers now and I massage their heads whenever I can. They are taller than I am, so I stand on a stool, or else they sit and I stand. As I massage their heads, they have their head on my heart the entire time. And that's an enormously wonderful feeling. They never take their head away from my chest until I tell them it's done. They know—they feel my love. There is no protest—they want to feel the love through a massage.

Another of our authors, Margaret Mullins, MSN/CFNP, recalls how she started massaging her daughters long before massage was popular in this country. *"When my twin daughters* [yes, both Margaret and Kumuda have twin daughters!] *were born twenty years ago, there was no information about baby massage available, except for one book, written by the famous French obstetrician Frederick Leboyer. His book described the traditional Vedic art of baby massage that he witnessed in his travels to India.*

"I tried massaging my daughters, and even though I had no training, I found that they responded with great pleasure. Even as they grew older, they insisted that I do it every night before bed. I also received many comments from other mothers on how well my daughters napped. Everyone wanted to know my secret for accomplishing this.

"A few years later, I became the director of the Mother and Baby program in Washington, D.C. It was fulfilling to be given specific information on how to do the massage in its most complete way, and to learn all the subtleties that are involved. Learning how to do the strokes, and the length of time to do them, is invaluable to new mothers."

Another mother, Lana, age 36, comments, *"Our new baby boy loves the oil massage and bath. He's incredibly healthy. His digestion is working better than our first child's at this age, and he doesn't have colic. He's all-around stronger, especially his muscle-tone. I think his robust health is partly because of the baby abhyanga and my diet, which is definitely better this time around, since I'm following the recommendations of the Mother and Baby program. I think the abhyanga is keeping his immune system strong. My older son has come home with colds from school many times and the baby doesn't get them. I'm really grateful."*

Karen Oelberg (introduced in Chapter Ten as a Mother and Baby program technician) says, "I *taught the baby abhyanga to the mother of twin babies. She was completely overwhelmed with her responsibilities. When I arrived at her home, the babies were screaming and needed bathing. The husband was going out to the gym and was leaving the whole mess behind. I took one baby and the mother took the other one. We put those babies on towels on the floor and they were crying and intense at the start. As soon as the oil touched them, they just relaxed and started to look as though they were on the beach in Hawaii—totally sprawled out. By the time we had them bathed they were radiant and ready for their naps.*

"It really transformed them, took the stress of birth off. It washed them clean inside and out. They were totally transformed. Normally there's a tension in newborns' bodies from the whole birthing process, and this was so soothing to them. They looked like totally different beings!

"If parents realized how this massage relaxes the baby, especially during the first months when digestive problems are common, they would take the time to do it. It would be much easier on the parents."

Fathers and Baby Massage

As for fathers, the baby abhyanga is something that the father can do just as well as the mother. Sometimes fathers feel excluded from the close relationship that mothers and babies form as a result of breast-feeding. That's why dads often claim the infant massage as their job. It gives them a chance to show their love in an active way, and it definitely helps bonding. If trained in baby abhyanga, fathers can learn how to get comfortable handling their fragile newborns—even when they're slippery with oil!

One father says, "*We had been married for eleven years before having children, so you can imagine that the first few weeks were a harrowing experience. Our daughter Candace was only about three weeks old when she had her first baby massage. She cried a little, kicked, and screamed. Then she seemed to relax and enjoy it. I picked her up after the massage, and she looked so fresh and radiant. She looked really relaxed, and fell asleep in my arms.*

"That was a turning point for me. It made me realize that I could survive, that having children could be quiet and comfortable too. The baby abhyanga seemed to turn our sweet-but-cranky, brand-new baby into a sweet-but-quiet brand-new baby. Having daily massages produced a dramatic change for her, very discernible. It made a big difference in my psychology. As a new father, I found it fun to have a baby."

Noreen, age 41, says, *"I hear that some babies have a hard time getting used to their bodies. I remember thinking that Michael seemed very comfortable in his body because of the baby abhyanga. It made him feel very relaxed and it brought him bliss. We have tapes of him being massaged and it's so beautiful. My husband would give him his massage. It's nice for the dad to be involved also, to enliven the connection between father and child. He would massage Michael's arms and you'd just see Michael's head going back in this ecstasy."*

A Review of New Baby Care

Here are some of the ways Maharishi Vedic Medicine suggests nourishing your child during the first six weeks.

- Protect your baby from crowds and the outside environment. While it is healthy to take your infant outside to breathe fresh air if the weather is mild, you will want to protect him or her from the elements.
- Avoid exposing your infant to any situations that might startle or frighten him. Don't toss the baby into the air (as parents sometimes do in fun) or leave the baby alone.
- Keep your baby warm.
- Give your child a daily abhyanga after the umbilical cord falls off.
- Follow the massage with a warm bath. (Until the umbilical cord falls off, Maharishi Vedic Medicine suggests giving a sponge bath.)

- Dress your child in fresh, clean, loose clothes.
- Avoid exposing your baby to harsh light, cold, drafts or direct wind, and loud sound.
- Keep your baby with you in a quiet room away from the main activity of the house until he or she is six weeks old. Try to limit visitors to a few hours a week. This will give both of you a chance to rest and bond with each other.
- Support the baby's neck and head at all times, as the bones are very tender. The neck should be supported until he is able to hold his head without bobbing.
- Playing Maharishi Gandharva Veda music at a soft volume can help create a soothing, harmonious atmosphere for the baby.

Summary

Giving your baby a daily abhyanga is an ideal way to help your baby develop emotionally, physically, and mentally. The massage helps to promote sleep, strengthens digestion, and helps the baby relax.

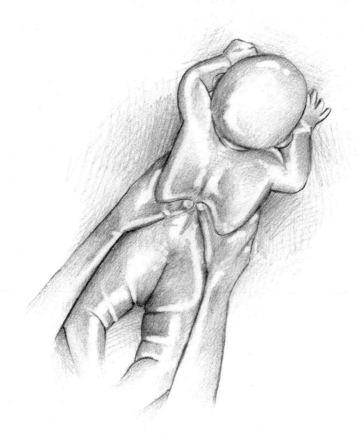

"Excessive anger, grief, and lack of maternal love, etc., result in suppression of lactation. In such cases, the woman should be cheered up and given a special diet in order to start the production of milk."
—*Sushruta Samhita*[75]

CHAPTER FIFTEEN

Breast-feeding, Weaning, and First Foods

For thousands of years, Ayur-Veda has noted that mother's milk is the ideal nourishment for the baby. Modern medicine has come to the same conclusion, and this is now the official recommendation of the American Academy of Pediatrics.

Mothers today breast-feed their babies because of the many emotional, physical, and mental advantages breast-fed children display as they grow up. The mortality rate for breast-fed infants is lower than the rate for bottle-fed ones. Studies have shown that mother's milk is ideal for the baby's digestion and contains all the nutrients your baby needs in an easily digestible form. (It even comes at the right temperature!) Breast-fed babies are said to have better immunity, and research shows that antibodies are transmitted in the mother's milk.[76]

Breast-fed babies have fewer psychological problems later in life. Perhaps this happens as a result of the love that is communicated when mothers nurse their children. Breast-feeding creates an intimate feeling between mother and child, which is essential for the child's future mental balance and happiness. It creates a protective and tender feeling in the mother, and helps establish the delicate bond of love.

Research on Breast-feeding

Not so long ago in this country, bottle-feeding became popular and only a small percentage of all mothers breast-fed, reaching an all-time low of 25 percent in 1970.[77] Since then, fortunately, mothers have begun to realize that breast-feeding is best for the child, and breast-feeding is again widely practiced in America.

Research on breast-feeding reveals a startling range of benefits. In a study of 383 Chicago children who were breast-fed, it was found that the breast-fed children were physically and mentally more developed than bottle-fed children. The bottle-fed were less nutritionally sound, got sick more often, and took longer to walk and talk. And the children who were breast-fed from four to nine months were more advanced than children who were only breast-fed for three months or less.[78]

Breast-feeding exercises the jaw and tongue, giving rise to more developed facial and dental structures, with less need for orthodontic repairs later in life.[79] Breast-feeding also provides the nutrients needed for healthier teeth and less cavities. It's interesting that dental decay is so much more prevalent among non-breastfed children that it is called the "nursing-bottle syndrome."

Even the development of speech is much more advanced in breast-fed children, probably because the same organs that are exercised and developed in breast-feeding are also used for speech. In a study that involved 319 children ages five or six, it was found that breast-fed children were superior in speech development, clarity of articulation, tonal quality, reading ability, and general confidence.[80]

Learning How to Breast-feed

Most women find that breast-feeding is very natural and enjoyable. However, even women who end up breast-feeding their child happily for many months may need some help getting started. Usually a nurse will help you with the first breast-feedings in the hospital, but with today's short hospital stays you may not be comfortable with it before you leave. That's perfectly normal. It could take a few days or weeks to get comfortable with the whole procedure. Don't be afraid to ask for help—it's important to get the help you need and feel relaxed with it as soon as possible.

There are several organizations to help you with free advice on breast-feeding, such as the La Leche League, which has support groups in most cities. Sometimes a clinic or hospital will send a nurse-consultant to your home to help you with breast-feeding during the first few weeks after giving birth.

It is essential for the mother to get enough rest if she wishes to nurse successfully. According to the Maharishi Vedic Approach to Health, breast-feeding takes even more strength than pregnancy. Also, many women find that breast-feeding is much more difficult if they are tense or nervous about doing it right.

It is usually easier to breast-feed if you are alone when you nurse, without distractions. Then you can focus on your baby and let your love flow with the milk. Give yourself time to adjust, and be patient with yourself. Also, practicing the Transcendental Meditation program regularly can help you to get needed rest and to feel more inner calm. Your baby will sense that and feel less tense, too. The soothing procedures of the Mother and Baby program and the Transcendental Meditation technique help you to rest, relax, and enjoy your new role as a mother more.

The Transcendental Meditation program reduces anxiety. One interesting study found that the Transcendental Meditation technique greatly reduces cortisol, a hormone that increases in large concentrations during stress and anxiety. In this study, lower cortisol levels were found in people while they practiced the Transcendental Meditation technique. This points to a state of rest that is deeper than ordinary relaxation. The decrease in cortisol during the Transcendental Meditation technique was the same as when falling asleep, even though the subjects remained alert.

This is indicates the unique state of restful alertness that occurs during the Transcendental Meditation program.

A meta-analysis conducted at Stanford University showed that the Transcendental Meditation program was significantly more effective in reducing anxiety than other forms of relaxation, including concentration, contemplation, and muscle relaxation.[81]

Karen Oelberg (introduced in Chapter Ten as a Mother and Baby program technician) recalls how she helped a new mother relax enough to enjoy breast-feeding. *"When I came into her home she and the baby were in a tizzy. It was her first child and she was having lots of trouble with breast-feeding. I said, 'Let's just give the baby to your husband, and we'll do the massage on you.' The next day she said, 'It's just like a miracle. The nursing went so much better—I was so much more*

⋞ L E S S   S T R E S S ,   L E S S   A N X I E T Y ⋟

Reduced Anxiety—Comparison of the *TM* Program with Relaxation Procedures

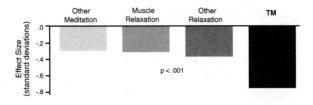

Reduction of Trait Anxiety

A statistical meta-analysis of all available studies (99 independent outcomes) indicated that the effect of the Transcendental Meditation program on reducing trait anxiety was approximately twice as great as that of all other meditation and relaxation techniques, including progressive muscle relaxation. Analysis showed that the positive result for the TM program could not be attributed to subject expectation, experimenter bias, or the quality of the research design.

This finding corroborates studies indicating that the TM technique produces substantially greater physiological effects than ordinary relaxation.

References: 1. K.R. Eppley, A.I. Abrams, and J. Shear, "Differential Effects of Relaxation Techniques on Trait Anxiety: A Meta-Analysis," *Journal of Clinical Psychology*, 45, (6) (1989). 2. M.C. Dillbeck, "The Effect of the Transcendental Meditation Technique on Anxiety Level," *Journal of Clinical Psychology*, 33 (1977), pp. 1076-1078.

---

relaxed and patient. Everything just switched after the massage.' Then I taught her how to massage her baby, too, and everything just relaxed. One of her friends, who had given her the Mother and Baby program as a gift, told me, 'She said you were like an angel sent from heaven. The massage was a real turning point for her.'"

Problems with Gas

You've probably seen mothers burping their babies and gently bouncing them when they seem fussy. That's because babies often have gas, caused because their delicate new digestive systems are not yet functioning perfectly. If some of the milk doesn't get digested properly, it causes pockets of air to collect in the digestive tract. Burping helps dispel the air pocket, as does bouncing.

Here are some other ways to help your baby digest better.

Daily Abhyanga: One of the best ways to help your baby's digestion is to give him an abhyanga each morning. This helps digestion and elimination. If your baby is fussy during the day, you can gently massage his tummy with warm sesame oil using a circular motion from right to left, for about nine circles. Then cover the tummy with a warm washcloth for five minutes. Placing a hot water bottle on your baby's stomach for ten to fifteen minutes can also help dispel gas. You'll want to purchase a baby-sized hot water bottle and make sure the water is not too hot.

Karen Oelberg remembers teaching the baby abhyanga to a mother whose baby was so colicky, it was a nightmare for her. "*I didn't teach her how to give her baby an abhyanga until later on, around three months, when the baby was almost at the end of the colicky period. But that baby just loved it, and it did cure his colic. Once when she didn't have time to do the abhyanga for a few days, the colic started coming back a bit, so she started up again. She told me she would just start to undress him and he would just go into ecstasy—he'd start waving his arms and get really happy because he'd know he was going to get his massage.*"

Baby Exercises: There are also "baby aerobics," or gentle stretching exercises, that you can do with your child for five minutes after the baby massage. These are fun to do—your baby will love them—and they also help digestion. You can get the instructions for the baby exercises from your physician at a Maharishi Ayur-Veda Health Center or Maharishi Vedic Medical Center.

Feeding on the Modified Demand Schedule: During the first two weeks you will just want to feed your baby whenever he or she is hungry. After that, Maharishi Vedic Medicine recommends that you try a "modified demand" schedule. This means feeding the baby whenever he or she is hungry, but not less than two hours after the last feeding. This is because it takes about two hours to digest the milk, and if you feed your baby more often, adding new milk on top of partially digested milk, it could cause gas.

Of course, you don't want to be rigid about this schedule, but it is good to realize that your baby may have reasons other than hunger for crying. (If your baby cries before the two hours have passed, check to see if a wet diaper is the problem.) Usually, mother and baby settle into a natural schedule within a few weeks.

Claire, age 47, mother of three boys, used a feed-on-demand schedule with her first child. *"With John I was really, really tired,"* she says. *"It was a tremendous adjustment, because he nursed all the time. He had such bad colic that I had to walk back and forth down the block just bumping him up and down to give him some relief. By evening he was just beside himself. I realize now that I was feeding him undigested milk on top of partially digested milk and he was getting heartburn and colic. And I didn't know this because I was told to feed on demand to keep the milk supply up.*

"With the second and third children, I used the recommendations of the Mother and Baby program, which meant that after the first two weeks you get them onto a two-hour feeding schedule. They didn't have any kind of colic or indigestion, and my milk came in regularly, too."

Dietary Recommendations and Herbal Supplements: As Chapter Fourteen described, by avoiding foods that cause you indigestion, you will help your baby's digestion, too. You'll want to follow the recommended diet and take the recommended herbal supplements.

Herbal Tea to Relieve Gas: One of the Maharishi Ayur-Veda herbal teas that is prescribed for postpartum mothers can be given directly to your baby by teaspoon when he or she feels fussy. Many mothers have found that giving their baby just a sip of the tea brings immediate relief.

One 31-year-old mother, Terri, says she used the Maharishi Ayur-Veda herbal tea with her daughter, who responded very quickly and easily. *"She really liked it. She often had a tummy ache in the evening—the tea seemed to reduce her discomfort quickly. She'd be crying and would stop as soon as she had the tea."*

Additional Problems

Keeping the breast milk healthy is a primary concern of Maharishi Vedic Medicine. Because the baby has such a delicate digestion, the milk must be healthy or the baby will get sick. The Mother and Baby program includes recommendations from *Charaka Samhita* and other Vedic texts, which describe how to keep the mother's milk rich, nutritious, and copious. There are recommendations for diet, herbs, and purification therapies to promote healthy milk and to help correct any problem with lactation caused by imbalance of the mother's doshas.

If you find that you are having difficulties with breast-feeding, then a physician/practitioner trained in Maharishi Vedic Medicine can determine which doshas need to be brought into balance and prescribe natural therapies to improve the quality and quantity of your milk. Usually, just following the general recommendations of the Mother and Baby program is enough, but if you are already following the program and the problem persists, be sure to consult your physician/practitioner.

Dry or cracked nipples: Sometimes mothers have trouble with their nipples drying out or cracking from frequent breast-feeding. The Mother and Baby program recommends applying ghee to the nipples prior to nursing. Ghee is nourishing for the baby and helps lubricate and protect the nipples during nursing. Applying a warm compress over the nipples before nursing is also comforting, as it brings increased blood and circulation to the area, which aids the healing capacity of the cells.

Blocked Milk Ducts or Insufficient Milk Flow: It helps to gently massage your breasts daily after the milk comes in, to prevent blocked milk ducts. Warm compresses are also helpful. Apply warm compresses to the breasts for four to five minutes before nursing, because the heat expands the tissues and helps the blocked area to drain. Once the baby is suckling well the massage and hot compresses are no longer necessary.

If for some reason there is not enough milk, the mother should make sure she is getting enough rest. Also, it is worth repeating that it is usually easier for the mother if she is alone when she nurses, without distractions. Then she can focus on her baby and let her love flow with the milk.

Unhealthy Milk: The Vedic texts describe in detail what healthy mother's milk should look and taste like. Unhealthy milk might not affect the mother's health, but because it is the child's sole means of nourishment and the child has a tender digestive system, it can cause abnormal stool, pain in moving bowels, constipation, thick urine, cramps, shivering, and inflammation of the nose, eyes, and mouth. The causes of unhealthy breast milk are an unwholesome or heavy diet, fasting, anger, grief, diseases, and breast-feeding one child while pregnant with another. Maharishi Rejuvenation therapy (panchakarma) and herbal supplements are strongly recommended, according to which doshas are out of balance. A physician trained in Maharishi Vedic Medicine can prescribe Maharishi Ayur-Veda herbal supplements and other treatments to restore balance to the mother's health.

Night Nursing: It's easier to nurse at night if the baby is in the same room with you for at least the first three months. (In India, babies are often even kept in the same bed with the parents.) This is also important for safety's sake, as you don't want to leave a newborn alone at night in case he chokes, gets a fever, or vomits during the night. After three months, if you feel the need to move him into another room, you can use a baby monitor to make sure you can hear any signs of discomfort.

It's good to stop middle-of-the-night feedings after your baby is six to nine months old because they increase congestion (imbalanced Kapha dosha) and disturb sleep patterns. Once the child starts eating solids, you can go longer between feedings. If your baby continues to wake up at night, you can offer water. Eventually he will get bored with having only water and will stop waking up.

Fear of Breast-feeding: Some mothers fear that their breasts will become permanently out of shape from breast-feeding. The good news is that breast-feeding actually helps the breasts to return to normal after pregnancy. Also, even though some people think that breast-feeding is too time-consuming, it is, in fact, more convenient than preparing a baby's bottle!

Weaning Your Baby

You'll want to check with your pediatrician for advice on weaning. According to Maharishi Vedic Medicine, when your baby's first tooth appears, this is a sign from nature that he is ready to eat solid foods. Usually this occurs around five or six months of age. Of course, some children are ready even before this time. If your baby is showing an interest and desire for the food around him, this is often a good sign that he's ready to start.

The main guidelines are to begin with foods that are very easy to digest, and to introduce only one food at a time. This will help prevent your baby's digestion from getting overloaded. If ama (the sticky waste product of undigested foods) starts to accumulate, it could lead to allergies. You can get a complete set of guidelines for introducing solid foods, as well as personal advice for your baby, from your physician/practitioner.

First Foods: A thin rice broth or thin dahl broth made from split mung beans is recommended to start. Then you can gradually make it thicker and creamier. Eventually you can add vegetables and fruits that your baby likes, and move into a regular routine of three meals a day. As the number of nursings decreases, you can add cow's milk in gradually increasing amounts. If your baby has trouble digesting cow's milk, check with your pediatrician. Often children can digest cow's milk better after twelve months, so you might wait until then to introduce it. Goat's milk is less nourishing but easier to digest, so you could try that during the transition time before your child is ready for cow's milk.

As you introduce the new foods, you'll continue breast-feeding, although your milk supply will naturally decrease as the baby eats more solids. It's better to keep breast-feeding for three months after you introduce the new food.

It's recommended that you avoid feeding your baby sour foods, such as strawberries, yogurt, cheese, and grapefruit. Bananas are heavy and can cause congestion, so you'll want to go light on those. Meat, fish, eggs, and other heavy foods are difficult to digest and thus are not recommended until after one year.

Maharishi Vedic Medicine recommends eleven months as the optimal age to wean your child. By then she will have enough teeth to chew, and will be accustomed to eating a solid diet. Continuing to breast-feed for a longer period of time can be exhausting to the mother, with fewer and fewer gains for the child. Also, many mothers report that it is emotionally easier for the child to be weaned at eleven months rather than fourteen months or later. The older she gets, the more she is aware of her surroundings, and the harder it may be for her to stop breast-feeding. However, you'll want to take your own child's needs into consideration, and use your own maternal instincts to make a decision.

Teething: Teething is a time when the child is susceptible to fevers and other diseases. It's interesting that the Vedic texts give detailed information about the time for teething and health of children's teeth, and how to treat various problems that can come up, including treatment of defective teeth and gums. Various symptoms can accompany teething (such as fever and indigestion), and your physician/practitioner can prescribe herbal compounds to help relieve these symptoms.

Eating, like breast-feeding, should be a happy time for the child, when you share love and warmth. In India, there is a tradition of taking the child out to the veranda to eat, to see the flowers and the sun at the noonday meal. In the evening, the mothers point out the stars and moon as their children eat. There are folk songs that the mother sings to her child, "See the stars at night, beautiful moon, beautiful stars, come and feed my baby." In this way the child is nourished not only through food but through love and attention, and also learns that he is connected to the cosmos, to all of nature around him. It is natural for mothers in every culture to sing to their children and make eating first foods an enjoyable and soothing time.

Summary

Breast-feeding is the most natural way to nourish your child. According to modern research breast-fed children tend to be better adjusted, have fewer infections and childhood diseases, and are more advanced in speech.

"The path of love is like the relationship between a child and the heart of his mother. As the child takes his first step towards his mother her heart swells. Her happiness radiates and reflects on the child, so that at each step he enjoys greater happiness, and this again reflects in the heart of the mother. The mother's joy increases and reaches its height when the child arrives in her arms and finds himself one with the mother's heart." —Maharishi Mahesh Yogi[82]

CHAPTER SIXTEEN

Bonding with Your Baby

During recent decades, there has been a great deal of research on the very delicate thread connecting parent and child in mutual affection, called "bonding." Bonding is an extremely important phenomenon. Researchers say that children who bond with their parents are healthier, happier, and more successful in later life. And parents who bond with their children are more affectionate, more confident, and happier as parents.

What causes a parent and child to connect in such an intimate way? Many researchers feel that the first hours after birth are the most critical in establishing this bond. That's why many mothers today are choosing to have natural births, with a minimum of drugs, so both they and their children can be alert and share the joy of the first few moments of life, establishing tender attachments at the time when both are most receptive.

Of course, sometimes unforeseen complications can force the mother into having a Caesarean section or to take drugs to induce labor or lessen pain. In these instances, it is still possible to have a joyous birth with an opportunity for bonding. The more a parent and child interact in an intimate way, the more chance there is for bonding to take place.

While "bonding" is a modern term, the concept is an integral part of the Mother and Baby program. Because the mind and body are so intimately connected, sharing tender bonds of love helps the child grow in health and happiness, and helps the mother feel nourished in her role as provider. Bonding is a natural result of the Mother and Baby program, because love flows naturally when the mother is more rested and the mother and baby are well cared for.

Also, the Maharishi Vedic Approach to Health naturally gives maximum opportunity for bonding by recommending that the mother enjoy deep rest and inner happiness through the practice of the Transcendental Meditation program. Natural childbirth, breast-feeding, and baby abhyanga (oil massage) also promote bonding. In some ways, promoting the fine feelings of love and tenderness between mother and child is the most important result of the Mother and Baby program.

Research on Bonding Reveals Mind-Body Connection

In the past thirty years, the relationship between mother and child has been the subject of hundreds of research studies. This research verifies a central principle of Maharishi Vedic Medicine: that the mind and emotions have a direct influence on health. Here we see that the child's feelings of well-being are completely dependent on receiving love from the mother.

Some significant findings reported by researchers:

- Mothers who are able to have more contact with their children immediately after birth display more love and affection for their babies throughout life.[83]
- Children who learn the most quickly and seem happiest are those who have bonded with their mothers after birth.[84]
- Infants who form healthy attachments with their mothers shortly after birth (called "early-bonding infants" in the scientific literature) become much more self-sufficient, outgoing, intelligent, and happy than children who were separated from their mothers immediately after birth and kept

in a hospital nursery except for feedings.[85]

- Mothers who bond with their infants early tend to be better mothers. They tend to feel more self-assured and relaxed when handling their infants, with no anxiety or awkwardness.

- Similar findings have emerged about fathers who bond early with their children.

- Bonding is both indicated and promoted by behaviors such as cuddling, kissing, prolonged eye contact, cooing, and speaking nourishing words in a nourishing tone of voice.

Bonding First Occurs in the Womb

Research suggests that attachment between mother and child starts long before birth—perhaps even with the first thought, "I'm going to have a baby!"[86] Mothers and infants who bond immediately at birth might be drawing on a communication system set up long before. Studies show that the unborn child can sense whether the mother loves or wants him. In fact, the mother's attitude toward her baby before the baby was born—how much she loved and wanted the baby—is the biggest factor in determining the child's subsequent emotional and physical health.[87]

The link between mother and child is so intimate that even the new child's sleeping patterns will reflect the patterns he learned from being connected with his mother in the womb. One fascinating research study found that pregnant women who were early risers tended to give birth to babies who rose early after they were born. Late-rising mothers gave birth to late-rising babies.[88]

Even the father bonds with his baby before birth. One study found that when a man spoke to his child in short, soothing phrases, the newborn was able to pick out the father's voice in a room during the first hour or two of life. If the child was crying, for instance, he would stop crying when he heard the familiar, soothing voice of his father.[89]

The First Hours after Birth

Newborn children cannot see far distances. Yet children only a few hours old can see their mothers' faces clearly at a distance of six to twelve inches.

Much of the research on bonding, which focuses on the first hours after birth, shows the importance of keeping the mother and child together as much as possible in the first hours after birth. A natural birth allows the mother and child to be alert and awake during the first hour. Most of this time can be spent together just experiencing the joy of holding and touching your newborn. If this is medically possible, it is the ideal. If the birth is a Caesarean, you can still see your baby soon after the birth. You will be sore and uncomfortable, but you can still share this precious time with your child.

As mentioned in Chapter Nine, Maharishi Vedic Medicine recommends a natural childbirth, when medically possible. It's best to try to arrange ahead of time to have the room dimly lit (as the baby's eyes are not accustomed to bright lights) and warm (to keep the baby's skin temperature from falling). It's also best to arrange that there be no interruptions or loud noises. It's better to work out the details of the first hours after birth with your obstetrician ahead of time. Nowadays, most hospitals understand the need for mother and infant to spend time together after delivery and allow time for it. But it's better to be sure by discussing your ideas in advance.

The Father's Role

It's just as important for the father to bond with the baby as for the mother. For one thing, the father's participation and support of the mother is the single most important factor in making her feel safe and happy—which in turn allows her to nourish her child. The father's support is essential to the mother's well-being, and thus the child's. The stronger the participation of all the members of the family, the stronger will be the family as a unit.

Recent studies show that what affects the father's sense of commitment to his family most is bonding with his child.[90] Fathers are also more likely to display affectionate behavior with their newborns—kissing, hugging, rocking, touching, and holding—if they have had early contact with their child. In other words, the sooner fathers were able to see their babies, the more interested and engrossed they were, and the more likely they were to touch, hold and play with their infant.[91]

The Role of Breast-feeding and Baby Abhyanga in Bonding

Abhyanga (discussed in Chapter Fourteen) and breast-feeding (discussed in Chapter Fifteen) are important aspects of Maharishi Vedic Medicine. While both have primary benefits in promoting physical health, they also nourish the delicate bonds that start developing the first time the mother touches her baby or looks into his eyes.

Breast-feeding and abhyanga are also helpful in strengthening ties when bonding has been delayed. Bonding is still taking place during the first three months after birth. If the bonding process has been slow, or if there has been any interruption in forming the attachment (for instance if the baby is premature and must be separated from the mother and placed in an incubator after birth), breast-feeding and massage give the mother a wonderful opportunity to interact with her baby and express all the love she feels in her heart.

How Breast-feeding Improves Bonding: Modern research shows that there is an interesting relationship between breast-feeding and bonding. Breast-feeding mothers tend to bond with their infants. The kind of holding, hugging, and communicating that comes with breast-feeding certainly helps strengthen the love between mother and infant.[92] And in cultures where breast-feeding is the norm, mother-child contact is indeed more intimate overall.[93]

It's interesting that the converse is also true. Mothers who bond with their babies earlier tend to enjoy breast-feeding more and tend to continue to breast-feed for a longer period of time.[94]

How the Baby Abhyanga Improves Bonding: The mother's bonding to her baby is the basis for the child's developing a sense of trust. As mentioned earlier, during the bonding process, mothers look into their baby's eyes, display affectionate behavior, and touch their infants often.[95] The abhyanga is a great way for both mothers and fathers to bond with their child, because it gives a wonderful opportunity for physical touch and all of these bonding behaviors.

Noreen, age 41, recalls the pleasure of giving her son a baby abhyanga: *"Abhyanga is a great way to convey the message of love, and it creates such a connection between parent and child. That is how a baby receives love—through touch. To communicate on that level of tender feeling tells the baby a lot in just five or ten minutes' time. It is a gift of love to the child. I feel that our son embodies love, and maybe the massage enlivened that in him."*

Spoiling the Baby?

In the first part of the twentieth century, many parents in America and England were taught to refrain from giving their infants too much love and affection for fear of spoiling the child. Even today you may still hear someone advise you not to cuddle your infant so much because it might spoil him.

The mind and body are very closely connected. In fact, every thought and emotion triggers different hormones and chemicals that affect your whole body. For example, anger weakens the immune system, while feelings of love strengthen it. Happy thoughts create happy cells.

It makes sense, then, that the love that you give to your baby creates positive biochemical changes in both you and your baby.

This is why Maharishi Vedic Medicine says that giving your baby love is as important as providing food. It's natural and easy to love your baby—unless stress or fatigue gets in the way. By following the natural recommendations in Part II, you can feel rested enough to enjoy your newborn and let your love flow uninhibited by fatigue or stress.

Actually, research shows that babies need love—expressed in the form of holding, kissing, rocking, and cooing—to survive.[96] And the more love they receive in the earliest days and months, the more loving adults they become. In fact, the kinds of relationships and attachments your baby forms in infancy create effects throughout life. There will be a time and a place for discipline later on, but infants need to be nurtured and loved without limit.

Without touch, babies cannot grow normally. Babies who are not touched enough have been found to be underweight and shorter than normal, and if the touch deprivation is severe enough, may even die. They show aggression and anger in later life.[97] Adults who were loved, touched, and listened to as babies tend to have better self-esteem. They also form closer, more loving, relationships, and have happier marriages and closer friendships.[98, 99]

Fortunately, the Mother and Baby program helps to remove the fatigue and depression that could get in the way of the flow of love. I find with my patients that when postpartum mothers are able to follow the simple recommendations set forth in these chapters, then bonding happens so effortlessly and blissfully that the new mother feels completely energized and nourished by her new baby. She spontaneously gives him all the love he needs. She falls in love.

Sharon, age 44 and a mother of three children, tells her experience of bonding with her son: *"With my first baby, I didn't have the Mother and Baby program, and I experienced extreme depression. Fortunately, with my second child, getting the extra rest and nourishment from the Mother and Baby program made a big, big difference. I felt a sense of unboundedness from my first treatment. I would look into Jason's eyes and completely lose awareness of the boundaries between us. I would feel almost a sense of dizziness—as if I were literally falling in love with my baby. He's four now and still I can look into his eyes at times and have that experience of unity. It's just like we're one. And I feel that there's this life force that's bigger than both of us. It's a very spiritual experience. I think it's because with him, I was following the principles of the Maharishi Vedic Approach to Health, and was much more rested and settled and clear and happy than with my first baby."*

Summary

Sharing the tender bonds of love is essential for the baby's growth and the mother's happiness. Having a natural childbirth, spending time together during the first hours after birth, staying rested, breast-feeding, and giving your newborn a daily abhyanga are all aspects of Maharishi Vedic Medicine that help increase the tender bond between mother and child.

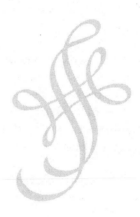

"If the child gets afflicted with any disease, he should be properly diagnosed, with due regard to the specific nature of the disease. Simultaneously, characteristic features of the patient, herbs, locality, season, and physical constitution of the child should be examined. Thereafter, he should be treated by administering therapies which are sweet, soft, light, fragrant, and propitious. Such types of therapies are wholesome for children and produce everlasting good effects.

"If he is free from any disease whatsoever, the child should be made to resort to regimens which bring balance to his individual constitution for the maintenance of positive health. Unwholesome regimens should be gradually changed to wholesome ones, and all things injurious for health should be avoided. By doing so, the child is endowed with excellent strength, complexion, physical constitution and span of life."   —*Charaka Samhita*[100]

CHAPTER SEVENTEEN

A Vision of Your Child's Future

As your baby grows into a child, you will naturally want to give all the attention and nourishment that he or she enjoyed as an infant. Fortunately, a major branch of Maharishi Vedic Medicine corresponds to our modern notion of pediatrics. This includes all of the various diseases of childhood and their treatments.

Because Maharishi Vedic Medicine cultivates not only the physical body, but the mind and emotions as well, it includes many recommendations for developing intelligence and contentment in children. The goal is to raise children without stress, who grow naturally in happiness, intelligence, and perfect health. While raising healthy children is the topic of another book, a few highlights are included here, just to give a glimpse of the possibilities.

Growing in Enlightenment

Maharishi Vedic Medicine aims to help every child develop his or her full potential. In fact, the Vedic ideal is for young people to reach the state of full human development—known as enlightenment—by the time they are twenty-five. This means they are then prepared for living in bliss, perfect health, and success. It means living a life free from mistakes—a harmonious, productive life in service to society. The programs of the Maharishi Vedic Approach to Health begin at birth and provide a variety of techniques to keep the mind and body perfectly balanced, so children grow into this state of full human development, or enlightenment, effortlessly and naturally.

From birth until age twenty-five, the most important influence on a child's life is the parents. Young children tend to reflect their environment, and parents make up the major portion of their environment. If each parent's attention flows from a very coherent consciousness, the child's consciousness will naturally respond to and begin to partake of that same coherence.

Children depend on their parents for growth. Therefore, it's essential that you, as parents, continue your own growth at a maximum pace, and maintain your own optimum health through Maharishi Vedic Medicine, especially through the Transcendental Meditation technique. When you are feeling blissful, happy, and rested, it will be easy to let your love flow to your children and to give them proper guidance. It will also be easier for them to pay attention to your guidance, to understand it, and to follow it. When love is flowing in a harmonious way, then automatically love flows back to the parent. This bond of love maintains the health of the child.

As a physician trained in Maharishi Vedic Medicine, when I see a child for treatment, I look first to the parents. Are they enjoying a healthy routine? Are they feeling blissful and stress-free? If there is an imbalance in the child, it often starts with an imbalance in the family structure itself. And often it is caused simply by the mother being tired.

After all, parents can only give from what they have. If they are a reservoir of bliss and positive feelings, this overflows to the child. Knowing how important it is to feel happy and healthy yourself, you can use the therapies of Maharishi Vedic Medicine to maintain balance in your family and let all that love flow through you.

Several research studies have shown how even the Transcendental Meditation program alone can improve your family life. One study from Canada (where health records are all maintained centrally) demonstrated how your family could enjoy reduced medical costs.

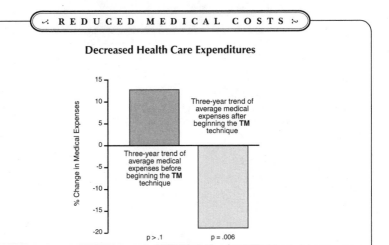

⌐ REDUCED MEDICAL COSTS ⌐

Decreased Health Care Expenditures

This chart shows three-year averages of medical expenses for physicians' services of participants before and after practice of the Transcendental Meditation program. In this study, government payments for physicians' services (approximately 20% of total medical expenses) were examined for 677 Quebec health plan enrollees who learned the Transcendental Meditation program. During the three years prior to beginning the Transcendental Meditation program, subjects' expenses (adjusted for inflation, age, and gender) did not change significantly. After learning the Transcendental Meditation program, subjects' adjusted expenses declined significantly, by 5-7% annually.

Reference: R.E. Herron, S.L. Hillis, J.V. Mandarino, D.W. Orme-Johnson, and K.G. Walton. "The Impact of The Transcendental Meditation Program on Government Payments To Physicians In Quebec," *American Journal of Health Promotion*, 10, (3) (1996), pp. 208-216.

Your children should be able to enjoy greater success in their schooling by practicing the Transcendental Meditation technique. Children as young as four years old can practice the Word of Wisdom technique[SM] and show tangible benefits. Like the

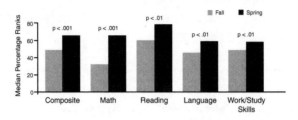

⤳ I M P R O V E M E N T S   A T   S C H O O L ⤺

Improved Performance on Iowa Test of Basic Skills

Within one academic year new students enrolled at Maharishi School of the Age of Enlightenment, where all students practice the Transcendental Meditation program, showed significant gains on the Iowa Test of Basic Skills, a nationally standardized test given to students in grades 1-8. Continuing students also made significant gains within one academic year (ref. 1). A second study (ref. 2) showed significant gains in grades 9-12 on the Iowa Test of Educational Development. A third study (ref. 3) found that the length of time students had been practicing the TM program was significantly correlated with academic achievement, independent of IQ scores.

References: 1. S.I. Nidich, R.J. Nidich, and M. Rainforth, "School Effectiveness: Achievement Gains at Maharishi School of the Age of Enlightenment," *Education,* 107 (1986), pp. 49-54.
2. S.I. Nidich and R.J. Nidich, "Student Academic Achievement at Maharishi School of the Age of Enlightenment," presented at the Midwest Educational Research Association (Chicago, IL, October 1986).
3. S.I. Nidich and R.J. Nidich, "Holistic Student Development at Maharishi School of the Age of Enlightenment: Theory and Research," *Modern Science and Vedic Science,* 1 (4) (1987).

Higher Level of Moral Reasoning

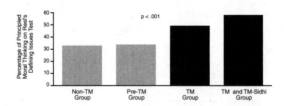

Students practicing both the Transcendental Meditation and TM-Sidhi programs scored the highest of four groups tested on degress of principled moral reasoning.

Reference: S.J. Nidich and D.W. Orme-Johnson, "Kohlberg's Stage Seven, Natural Law, and the *Transcendental Meditation* and *TM-Sidhi* Programs," *Proceedings of the International Symposium of Moral Education* (Fribourg, Switzerland, September 3, 1982).

adult TM technique, the Word of Wisdom technique is a simple, effortless technique, but practiced for a reduced amount of time with eyes open. One study on four-year-olds practicing this technique found that over a six-month period they exhibited significant acceleration in their cognitive development and intelligence measures.[101]

Other studies have found that elementary and secondary school students practicing the Transcendental Meditation program demonstrate improved academic achievement and greater maturity in their moral reasoning.

Several researchers in different countries have studied the ef-

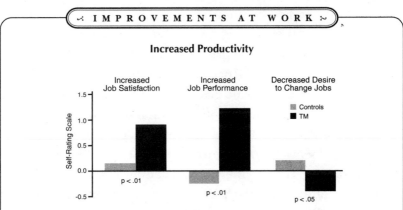

IMPROVEMENTS AT WORK

Increased Productivity

Subjects at all levels of responsibility in business practicing the Transcendental Meditation program for an average of 11 months showed significant improvements at work compared with nonmeditating members of a control group. Relationships with co-workers, supervisors, and family members also improved. The degree of these improvements increased as the subjects continued practicing the TM technique.

References: 1. D.R. Frew, "*Transcendental Meditation* and Productivity," *Academy of Management Journal*, 17 (1974), pp. 362-368.
2. K.E. Friend, "Effects of the Transcendental Meditation Program on Work Attitudes and Behavior," in D.W. Orme-Johnson and J.T. Farrow (editors), *Scientific Research on the Transcendental Meditation Program: Collected Papers, Vol. 1* (Livingston Manor, NY: MERU Press, 1977), pp. 630-638.
3. C.N. Alexander, G. Swanson, M. Rainforth, T. Carlisle, and C. Todd, "The Effects of the Transcendental Meditation Program on Stress Reduction, Job Performance, and Health in Two Business Settings," presented at the National Conference of the Center for Management Research, Maharishi International University (Fairfield, IA, May 23, 1987).

fects of the Transcendental Meditation technique on productivity and relationships at work. Not too surprisingly, the decreased stress and broader awareness have produced some remarkable results.

Maintaining a Good Routine

Probably the most important advice I can give to parents is to put yourselves and your children on a good daily routine, so that your rising time, bedtime, and eating habits are all in tune with nature. When parents and children stay rested, many health problems clear up or never even arise. Here are some of the recommendations from Maharishi Vedic Medicine:

1. **Go to bed early.** The foundation of a healthy routine for children is to get them to bed early. Resting when nature is resting and getting enough sleep are essential to good health. Lack of rest is often the precursor to a cold or other sickness.
2. **Wake up with the sun and give your child a daily abhyanga.** The oil massage helps develop the brain and central nervous system of infants. As children get older, they can be taught to massage themselves to improve immunity and health.
3. **Practice the Transcendental Meditation technique with your whole family before school or work, and again in the early evening.** Children ten years and older can learn to meditate just like adults. Younger children learn a modified technique more suited for their young nervous systems, which they can do while they're active. Research shows that the Transcendental Meditation technique improves family relationships, mental and physical health, and intelligence. Families who meditate together grow in harmony together.
4. **Eat a light breakfast, and if possible, make the noon meal the largest meal of the day.** This is because the digestion is strongest at midday. If the children can come home for lunch, it's ideal to prepare a fresh, hot meal. Try to include all six tastes— sweet, sour, salty, pungent, bitter, and astringent—in every meal.

Eat a lighter evening meal, because food is harder to digest at night.

5. **Try to create a settled atmosphere before bed.** A quiet time of reading, listening to music, singing, or visiting is best. Maharishi Gandharva Veda music is especially settling. It's better to avoid stimulating mental activities, including watching too much television, right before bed.

If your whole family is living in tune with the clock of nature by following a healthy routine, then you'll find that life will grow increasingly balanced and blissful.

Seasonal Check-ups

Children, like adults, have their own unique make-up, and need to eat the foods and follow a daily routine that will help their own individual nervous systems stay in balance. If you bring your children to a Maharishi Ayur-Veda Health Center for seasonal check-ups, then you can find out the most suitable foods, routines, and other recommendations for your child.

Some children, for example, may be more prone to rashes, tender skin, and impulsiveness. These children may have more Pitta dosha, and will do better if they avoid eating hot, spicy foods. Another child may have trouble falling asleep at night or may be thin for her height. She may need a diet and daily routine to balance Vata dosha.

If your children receive seasonal check-ups, your physician/practitioner can help keep the doshas in balance and prevent disease before it starts. Think of how much easier life would be if your children didn't get sick as often!

The Vedic texts are astonishingly thorough in describing the diagnosis and treatment of dozens of childhood ailments. In fact, pediatrics is a highly developed branch of Maharishi Vedic Medicine, and there are many natural treatments to keep children healthy, including dentistry.

Vegetarian Diet

Although it is not necessary to be a vegetarian to enjoy the benefits of the Maharishi Vedic Approach to Health, a vegetarian diet is recommended because there are many advantages to not eating meat.

Modern research has begun to report significant evidence that vegetarian diets are healthier. For instance, vegetarians have a lower rate of colon cancer and certain other cancers. According to the American Cancer Society, up to thirty-five percent of new cancer cases could be avoided by following proper dietary recommendations. Obesity, gall bladder disease, hypertension, and adult diabetes are found less often in those following a vegetarian diet. Also, vegetarians have lower cholesterol, which is a major risk factor in the development of cardiovascular disease.

If you and your family are currently eating meat on a regular basis, you might want to start by reducing the number of meals that include red meat. You could eat poultry or fish instead. These are easier to digest.

Over time, you can reduce the number of meals with poultry and fish, and eat vegetarian meals more often. Discuss with your physician how to make sure you and your children are getting enough protein.

Whatever foods you eat, it's important not to strain. Enjoy your food, and eat more of the foods you know are healthy. As you follow the recommendations of Maharishi Vedic Medicine, you'll find that your mind and body are more in tune with nature, and you'll naturally enjoy the foods that are good for you.

Family Planning

Once you have one child, the joy and happiness you experience may naturally inspire you to have another. Maharishi Vedic Medicine recommends that the ideal time between pregnancies is from three to four years. The mother needs time for her physiology to recover and recuperate. This also gives the mother a chance to focus on one child at a time and give the child all the nourishment and care he or she needs.

The World is My Family

Parents have the responsibility to stay rested, happy, and healthy to be able to give more to their children. If parents are happy, children will be happy. As they welcome new children into the family, the parents must be sure to keep the bond of love between them lively, as children thrive on the love of their parents.

One father reports, *"With our whole family enjoying the recommendations of the Maharishi Vedic Approach to Health, we've experienced a wonderful feeling of well-being, perfect health, and harmony growing within our family.*

"Our daughters (ages 14 and 16) get to bed early, so naturally they wake up happier. They understand that if you sleep well, you feel better the next day.

"If the girls are coming down with something, or feel run down, they do an abhyanga and feel fresher. By taking rest when it's needed, they don't get sick. The abhyanga especially helps my younger daughter. She is very goal-oriented, very achievement-oriented, very active, and she has a predominance of Pitta and Vata. She doesn't believe in obstacles, which is great, but this tremendous drive needs to be mellowed out sometimes. Daily abhyanga was prescribed when she was four or five, and it still works. All the stress and tension just falls away—she turns into a ball of mush, a love bug. It makes a huge difference in her personality. It washes away the irritability.

"When my older daughter takes Maharishi Amrit Kalash herbal supplements, she's less likely to get colds. Now that she's entered her teenage years, she's also emotionally happier if she takes Rejuvenation for Women, a special herbal compound. It tends to balance her moods.

"And we all practice the Transcendental Meditation program together,

which my wife and I feel has made us all much closer and happier as a family. We are pleased that our children want to contribute to a more peaceful world by meditating every day to help create more harmony in themselves, our family, and our world family."

It is so important for children to experience happiness and bliss, and for parents to do everything they can to structure an orderly, harmonious environment so that children don't make wrong choices and suffer from their mistakes. If children are happy and healthy, then naturally as they grow older, their happiness will expand to include their family, community, profession, the world, and the whole universe.

This is the true meaning of the Vedic expression *vasudhaiva kutumbakam*—"The world is my family." Maharishi Vedic Medicine provides an approach to parenting that seeks to produce children who are living in tune with natural law, children who feel as much beautiful love for everything in creation as they do for their own selves.

Summary

The natural principles of Maharishi Vedic Medicine can be enjoyed by every member of the family, to develop the full potential of every child and to raise family life to the loving, joyful expression of Heaven on Earth.

APPENDIX

The Vedic Approach to Common Concerns During Pregnancy

As your body changes to accommodate your growing baby, you may notice some aches, pains, and general discomfort at times. While these are usually minor, you will want to check with your primary care physician if they come up.

Your physician/practitioner trained in Maharishi Vedic Medicine may also have some natural, simple solutions to these irritating and uncomfortable symptoms. Here are a few examples:

Muscle Cramps

Early in pregnancy there are many changes in nutrition and circulation, and as the blood and nutrition are directed toward the fetus, some women start to experience bodily changes. Muscle cramps often occur during the first trimester. This usually happens in the lower legs and calves.

To relieve the pain, massage calves with warm sesame oil and follow with a warm bath. Gentle stretching exercises, such as Yoga asanas, also can help.*

Straightening your legs and flexing your toes slowly toward

---

*To learn Yoga asanas, you can take a course on Maharishi Yoga at a Maharishi Vedic University, School, or Center, or at a Maharishi Ayur-Veda Health Center or Maharishi Vedic Medical Center. See Appendix C for more information.

your face can also help relieve the pain. To prevent muscle cramping, be sure you are eating a balanced diet with plenty of calcium. You can also try putting your feet up at intervals when engaged in physical activity.

If the pain continues, be sure to consult your doctor to make sure a blood clot is not forming.

Backache

Sometimes the enlarging uterus creates pressure on the sciatic nerve, causing pain in the buttocks and legs as well as the lower back. It's possible for the position of the baby to change, but in some cases the pain will continue throughout pregnancy.

This can be remedied by stretching exercises such as Yoga asanas. (Practicing these regularly can be a great *prevention* technique, too.) It also helps to lie on your back and lift your legs thirty to thirty-five inches while stretching and pointing your toes. A back massage can also help soothe and dissolve muscular tension. In severe cases, your doctor may recommend a few days of bed rest.

Puffy Feet

Swelling of the feet and ankles (edema) occurs at some time during pregnancy for the majority of women, due to circulation problems that often accompany pregnancy. You might notice your feet swelling in hot weather or after you have been sitting or standing for a long time. Interestingly, drinking more water actually helps, because it flushes out impurities and helps relieve water retention.

You can also soak ten to fifteen black raisins in water for six to eight hours. Eat the raisins and drink the water. Repeat twice a day. It also helps to take walks to improve circulation, rather than lying in bed. Stretching exercises such as Yoga asanas also help. You can place pillows under your feet when you lie down, to relieve the discomfort. Often after resting for the night, the problem disappears.

If swelling persists or is serious, then contact your primary care obstetrician immediately.

Heartburn, Flatulence (gas), Indigestion, Nausea, and Morning Sickness

These problems are often caused by eating hard-to-digest foods, such as leftovers, meats, aged cheeses, and processed foods. Also, the expanding uterus pressing against your intestines doesn't help digestion much! The solution is to eat foods that are nourishing yet easy to digest, as recommended by your physician/practitioner (described in Chapter Six).

If the problem continues, take a little powdered ginger plus a pinch of rock salt. Eat it plain or add ½ teaspoon of lemon in a glass of water. This will stimulate your appetite if you eat it before the meal.

Or take a mixture of fresh lemon juice, water, and ginger juice. To a small glass of water, add ½ teaspoon freshly squeezed lemon juice. Add ½ teaspoon of fresh ginger juice to the lemon-water mixture. (You can make ginger juice by pureeing fresh ginger root in a blender or juicing it in a juicer.) Add two to three pinches of rock salt, and two to three pinches of natural sugar for flavoring. Sip it when you feel the need.

Also, you'll want to help your digestion by eating in a settled, quiet place without distractions. If you gulp your food and jump up after you eat, it can cause digestive disturbances.

Constipation

Constipation is a common problem, partly because the pressure of the growing fetus on your bowels makes them more sluggish. Also, hormonal changes due to pregnancy slow down elimination. That's why eating fresh, easily digestible foods is so important.

Include more whole grains and fresh fruits and vegetables, as the fiber content helps elimination.

Constipation is also due to internal dryness, so make sure you sip water with your meals and at bedtime, and be sure to drink at least eight glasses a day, preferably warm water. Drinking a cup of water that has been left standing in a copper vessel overnight can help to relieve constipation as well. As mentioned under "Puffy Feet," it's also helpful to soak ten to fifteen black raisins in water and eat them twice a day (drink the water they were soaked in, too).

Stuffy Nose

This complaint is a common one for pregnant women, and can even be accompanied by nosebleeds. While the nosebleeds can be caused by high levels of estrogen and progesterone, which cause the delicate mucous membranes of the nose to soften and swell, the stuffy nose is most likely to be caused by weak digestion and an accumulation of ama, the sticky waste-product of undigested food.

Drinking too many cold drinks and eating leftovers and processed foods can cause congestion. If you eat warm, freshly cooked foods, you will probably notice that this problem disappears. You can also take a pinch of turmeric and a pinch of black pepper and boil it in a cup of milk. Drink the milk warm. This helps relieve congestion.

There are also special herbalized oils to clear impurities from the sinuses. These also lubricate the inside of your nose and give immediate relief from dryness. (See Appendix C for ordering information.)

Summary of Research on Mother and Baby Program Participants

Ragnhild Boes, a Danish psychologist, conducted a study, *"Maternal Adjustment After Childbirth: An Investigation of the Effects of the Mother and Baby Program and the* TM *and* TM-Sidhi *Programs on Mothers' Postpartum Recovery,"* in partial fulfillment of the requirements for her Ph.D. in Psychology at Maharishi University of Management, Fairfield, Iowa.

Boes examined qualitative data from interviews with 31 women in Fairfield, Iowa, who gave birth between February 1993 and December 1995. Eighteen women, average age 34.5 years, participated in the Transcendental Meditation and TM-Sidhi programs, including Yogic Flying, and the *Maharishi Ayur-Veda* Mother and Baby program (Group I or "program" mothers), while 13 women, average age 27.7 years, did not participate in any of these three programs (Group II or "comparison" mothers). Interviews were conducted six and twelve weeks postpartum on five topics: family relationships; mother's emotional and bodily changes; health; energy level; and quality of sleep. Boes found major changes in family relationships, emotional and bodily changes, and health. Smaller changes were seen in energy levels and quality of sleep. The most striking finding was the greater overall stability in postpartum adjustment exhibited by "program" mothers in all the areas studied, both in their descriptions and in the percentages of categories covered by their reports.

Boes found that "program" mothers described their experiences of family relations, emotional/bodily stability and strength, energy level, confidence and happiness, and overall health in warmer, more positive terms. Although descriptions of energy level and quality of sleep indicated only small differences between groups over time, Boes found these differences to be especially noteworthy because the "program" mothers were significantly older (by 6.8 years) than the "comparison" mothers. Forty-four per cent of the "program" mothers were age 35 to 45 years, and a strong majority, 78%, were first-time mothers, which adds dramatic validation of the Mother and Baby program's benefits. The following are some highlights from her findings:

Family Relationships

"Program" mothers' reports of enriched family life were warmer and remained more consistent, more stable, than "comparison" mothers. Half of the "program" mothers described enriched family lives in happy, loving terms both at week 6 and at week 12, while the "comparison" mothers rated their family relations less positively and with greater variation between the two interviews.

At week six, enriched family life characterized by love, harmony, and sweetness was described by twice as large a proportion of "program" mothers as contrasted to "comparison" mothers (50% versus 25%).

At week 12 it was found that family cooperation and closeness in both groups had remained at about the same level as at week 6, and that reports of "having less time as a couple" were replaced by the experience of "having less time for other family members" because the baby takes more time. This change may be indicative of a shift from couplehood to familyhood, noted by mothers in both groups. While "program" mothers remained stable in terms of descriptions of enriched family life during this 6-week time period, the "comparison" mothers did not report enriched family life at week 12. Their family lives were characterized by more fluctuations—more ups and downs over time—and more stressful experiences.

Enriched Family Relations and Family Closeness

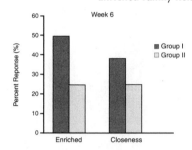 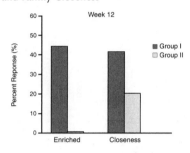

Descriptions of experiences with the Mother and Baby program

Some descriptions were as follows: "I felt prepared to start taking care of the family," commented a young, first-time mother. She also reported that "It is really good to have that time every day (for the Mother and Baby program). I would feel to give more to my family because I had time for myself."

"After the Mother and Baby program I would feel refreshed and really full of love," commented a young, first-time mother, while a mother of two children described how "The Mother and Baby program allows for us to stay cohesive as a family."

Emotional and Bodily Changes

In general, "program" mothers indicated emotionally and physically stabilizing and balancing results of the Mother and Baby program. Their reports of emotional strength, stability and comfort remained stable over time, while "comparison" mothers' reports indicated a more fluctuating, less enhanced quality of emotional well-being. Similarly, "program" mothers' reports of "confidence/happiness" remained stable from week 6 to week 12, while "comparison" mothers did not report confidence/happiness. Also, among the "program" mothers, those who participated longer in the Mother and Baby program gave more consistent de-

Emotional Stability and Confidence

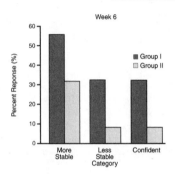 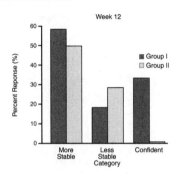

scriptions of feeling emotionally and stable, strong, and comfortable.

Descriptions of experiences with the Mother and Baby program

"Right away the first day . . . it was such a deep level—all those tensions and worries seemed to disappear. It is very helpful emotionally to stabilize. It has helped feeling happier and more cheerful," said a mother with two children.

"It gave me a lot more evenness—emotionally. I felt less moody, more comforted," commented a young first-time mother.

A first-time mother of more mature age said, "It helped me come into greater balance—physically and emotionally."

Another young, first-time mother told us, "I did not experience that postpartum depression, and I really think it had a lot to do with that."

"I felt fatigued and overwhelmed the first week. The Mother and Baby program took the edge off," said a mature, first-time mother.

"After the six weeks, I felt prepared to start taking care of the family, really taking on everything myself. I feel like I was really prepared to take care of everything—had time to think about it, get ready for it on a mental and emotional level. So now it is not a strain at all," commented a young, first-time mother.

"It gave me a good start for being a mother," said another young, first-time mother.

"It has made it possible for me to be a much better mother for my new baby and also for the other two," described a mother of two children.

"As I became more settled, more easy, he (the baby) also did. We just started to click together," was the experience of a new, first-time mother.

Health

A noteworthy difference between the two groups is that "pro-

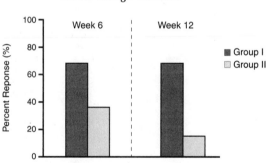

Health Ratings "Excellent"

gram" mothers' health ratings and descriptions remained stable over time at a higher level compared to "comparison" mothers, even though "program" mothers were an average of 6.8 years older.

Descriptions of experiences with the Mother and Baby program

"The Mother and Baby program is what helped me recover so quickly. It gave me the rest needed to recover properly," reported a young, first-time mother.

"That deep rest allowed me to bounce back to my state of health," reported another.

"It created a cushion of comfort—to get back to a natural state," commented a first-time mother over the age of 40.

"It has helped me get back to normal, it facilitates recovery," commented another young, first-time mother.

Energy Level and Quality of Sleep

While differences between the two groups were not great in these final two areas, the stability of "program" mothers' energy ratings and quality of sleep from week 6 to week 12 was notable, given their average age of 6.8 years older than the "comparison" mothers.

Information Sources on Maharishi Vedic Medicine and Related Programs

MAHARISHI VEDIC UNIVERSITIES, COLLEGES, SCHOOLS, AND CENTERS

Maharishi Vedic Universities, Colleges, Schools, and Centers are located in most major cities in the United States and in Canada. If you are unable to find a listing from your local telephone directory, or from directory assistance, call toll-free 888-532-7686, or see the following web site: http://www.Maharishi.org

Short Courses for the Whole Population
1. The *Transcendental Meditation* Program
2. Human Physiology: Expression of Veda and the Vedic Literature (Discovery under Maharishi's Guidance by Prof. Tony Nader, M.D., Ph.D.)
3. Good Health through Prevention
4. The *Maharishi Yoga* Program
5. Self-Pulse Reading Course for Prevention
6. Diet, Digestion and Nutrition

These courses are available at all Maharishi Vedic Universities, Colleges and Schools (see above). Full descriptions of these courses can be found at the same web site:
http://www.Maharishi.org

DEGREE PROGRAMS

Bachelor's degree program in Maharishi Vedic Medicine and doctoral degree program in Physiology with specialization in Maharishi Vedic Medicine:

Maharishi University of Management   515-472-1150
College of Maharishi Vedic Medicine
Fairfield, IA 52557
E-mail: admissions@mum.edu
Web site: http://www.mum.edu/cmvm

Two-year doctor training program; A.A. degree available for beginning students (curriculum authorized by the Commission on Higher Education for the Board of Education for the State of New Mexico):

Maharishi College of Vedic Medicine   505-830-0415
2721 Arizona Street, NE   fax: 505-830-0538
Albuquerque, NM 887110
E-mail: MCVMNM@aol.com

HOW TO LOCATE A PHYSICIAN
TRAINED IN MAHARISHI VEDIC MEDICINE

Contact your nearest Maharishi Vedic University, College, School, or Center (see above).

To contact Kumuda Reddy, M.D.:

1537 Union Street   518-377-0772
Schenectady, NY 12309

or

The Rainbow Healing Arts Center   914-229-8977
558 Albany Post Road (Route 9)
Hyde Park, NY 12538

Web site: http://www.allhealthyfamily.com

HOW TO LOCATE A TEACHER OF THE
TRANSCENDENTAL MEDITATION TECHNIQUE

Call toll-free 888-LEARN-TM (888-532-7686)
or see web site: http://www.tm.org

WHERE TO ORDER
MAHARISHI AYUR-VEDA HERBAL FORMULAS

In the United States

Maharishi Ayur-Veda Products	800-255-8332 or
International, Inc.	719-260-5500
P.O. Box 49667	
Colorado Springs, CO 80949-9667	
Web site: http://www.mapi.com	

In Canada

Maharishi Ayur-Veda Products Canada	800-461-9685 or
P.O. Box 9402	819-835-5485
40 Cochrane Road	
Compton, Quebec J0B 1L0	
Web site: http://www.all-veda.com	

CENTERS OFFERING THE
MAHARISHI REJUVENATION PROGRAM

In the United States

The Raj	800-248-9050 or
Fairfield, Iowa	515-472-9580
Web site: http://www.theraj.com	
Maharishi Ayur-Veda Medical Center	800-290-6702 or
Lancaster, Massachusetts	978-365-4549

In Canada

Maharishi Ayur-Veda College	800-575-5472 or
Compton, Quebec	819-835-5472
E-mail: cvmaha@sympatico.ca	
Maharishi Ayur-Veda Health Center	705-635-9041
Huntsville, Ontario	
Maharishi Ayur-Veda College	613-565-2030
Paterson House, Ottawa, Ontario	

More information is available at web sites:
http://www.Maharishi-medical.com
http://www.vedic-health.com

RECOMMENDED BOOKS

Books by Maharishi Mahesh Yogi

Life Supported by Natural Law. Washington, D.C.: Age of Enlightenment Press, 1986.

Maharishi Forum of Natural Law and National Law for Doctors. India: Age of Enlightenment Publications, 1995.

Maharishi Mahesh Yogi on the Bhagavad-Gita: A New Translation and Commentary, Chapters 1-6. New York: Penguin Books, 1973.

Maharishi Vedic University: Introduction. India: Age of Enlightenment Publications, 1995.

Science of Being and Art of Living. New York: Penguin Books, 1995.

Scientific Research on Maharishi Ayur-Veda Health Care

Scientific Research on Maharishi's **Transcendental Meditation** *and* **TM-Sidhi** *Program: Collected Papers,* Volumes 1-6, available through Maharishi University of Management Press, Press Distribution, DB 1155, Fairfield, Iowa 52557.

Scientific Research on the **Maharishi Transcendental Meditation** *and* **TM-Sidhi** *Programs: A Brief Summary of 500 Studies.* Fairfield, Iowa: Maharishi University of Management Press, 1996.

Other Books

Nader, Tony, M.D., Ph.D. *Human Physiology: Expression of Veda and the Vedic Literature.* The Netherlands: Maharishi Vedic University Press, 1994.

Denniston, Denise. *The* **TM** *Book: How to Enjoy the Rest of Your Life.* Fairfield, Iowa: Fairfield Press, 1986.

Marcus, Jay. *The Crime Vaccine: How to End the Crime Epidemic.* Baton Rouge, Louisiana: Claitor's Publishing Division, Inc., 1996.

O'Connell, David, and Charles N. Alexander. *Self Recovery: Treating Addictions Using* **Transcendental Meditation** *and* **Maharishi Ayur-Veda.** New York: Haworth Press, 1994.

Roth, Robert. *Maharishi Mahesh Yogi's* **Transcendental Meditation.** New York: Donald I. Fine, 1994.

Sharma, Hari, M.D. *Freedom from Disease: How to Control Free Radicals, a Major Cause of Aging and Disease.* Toronto: Veda Publishing, 1993.

Wallace, R. Keith. *The Neurophysiology of Enlightenment.* Fairfield, Iowa: Maharishi International University Press, 1986.

Wallace, R. Keith. *The Physiology of Consciousness.* Fairfield, Iowa: Maharishi International University Press, 1993.

These books and others are available from
Maharishi University of Management Press   800-831-6523
Press Distribution DB 1155
Fairfield, Iowa 52557
E-mail: mumpress@mum.edu
Web site: http://www.mum.edu/press

A selection of books is also available from Maharishi Ayur-Veda Products (see information above).

OTHER ASPECTS OF THE *MAHARISHI VEDIC APPROACH TO HEALTH* PROGRAM

Maharishi Gandharva Veda *Music*

Maharishi Gandharva Veda music is the classical music of the ancient Vedic civilization, the eternal rhythms and melodies of nature. It comes from the same age-old tradition of Vedic knowledge as Maharishi Ayur-Veda health care.

Like Ayur-Veda, the knowledge of Gandharva Veda music was restored to its original purity and completeness in this generation by Maharishi Mahesh Yogi. The purpose of this music is to neutralize stress in the atmosphere and create a harmonizing and balancing influence for the individual and society as a whole.

About Gandharva Veda music, Maharishi has explained, "Every level of creation is a frequency. One frequency melts into the other and this is how the process of evolution takes place. The night comes to an end and the dawn begins. At dawn, when the darkness and dullness of the night is over, some inspiring freshness comes and there is a different frequency in the whole atmosphere. At midday, there is another big change in frequency; at evening, a different frequency; at midnight, a different frequency. This cycle of change is perpetual, and because everything is a frequency there is sound at every stage.

"From morning to morning the melody of nature is changing. Gandharva music goes with the time, setting its melodies according to the changing nature. It sets forth those very natural melodies which match with the process of evolution. It provides a powerful harmonizing influence in the whole atmosphere to balance imbalances in nature.

"Gandharva music is the eternal melody of nature spontaneously sung in all levels of creation, from the most minute to the huge, enormous, ever-expanding universe. Gandharva Veda music creates a powerful melody from morning to morning, neutralizing the negative trends and tendencies born of the violation of natural law by the whole population of the world."

Maharishi Gandharva Veda music is available for all 24 hours of the day and night, on audiotape, videotape and compact disk. More information and samples of music can be heard on the internet at http://www.Maharishi.org

Additional information on Maharishi Gandharva Veda music products can be obtained from Maharishi Ayur-Veda Products, above.

The Maharishi Vedic Astrology *and* Maharishi Yagya *Programs*

The Maharishi Vedic Astrology program—the Vedic science of prediction—is another aspect of Maharishi Vedic Medicine. This knowledge has been applied from time immemorial to help foresee dangers that have not yet come.

Our immediate environment is our home, our neighborhood,

our city, country, continent and planet. Our extended environment is the universe around us—other planets, the sun, stars and distant galaxies. The Maharishi Vedic Astrology program, also called the Maharishi Jyotish^{SM} program, deals with this distant environment. Through a Maharishi Vedic Astrology consultation we can identify influences coming to us from our cosmic environment and take proper precautions to avert any negative effect.

The human physiology is part of the cosmic physiology. Every rhythm of the universe naturally has an effect on the individual, and vice versa. From the Maharishi Jyotish tradition we have the knowledge of how we interact with our cosmic counterparts.

Maharishi Jyotish knowledge becomes complete with the Maharishi Yagya program. A Maharishi Yagya performance is a precise action based on ancient Vedic wisdom and tradition that restores balance in the functioning of natural law. A Maharishi Jyotish consultation alerts you to a problem, but does not solve it. Maharishi Yagya procedures generate positive influences that restore the synchrony between individual rhythms and the rhythms of the cosmos.

As part of a Maharishi Vedic Astrology consultation, you receive recommendations for any necessary Maharishi Yagya performances to help avert a danger or to enhance the success of an undertaking. Influences that may favor diseases, accidents, lack of success in business, disharmony in marriage or any other problem can be minimized or avoided. A Maharishi Yagya procedure, performed before the danger arises, helps to neutralize negative influences so they do not reach you, and life remains in accord with natural law. Maharishi Yagya procedures may also be performed to enhance good periods in life and bring greater success, prosperity, and happiness.

For more information on the Maharishi Vedic Astrology and Maharishi Yagya programs:

In the United States

Maharishi Vedic Astrology program   800-888-5797

Maharishi Vedic Astrology and   515-472-5603
   Maharishi Yagya programs
Fairfield, Iowa

Maharishi Yagya program   603-588-4235
Antrim, New Hampshire
E-mail: MaharishiYagyaProgram@compuserve.com
Web site: http://www.Maharishi.org

Canadians: Contact the Maharishi Yagya program international office at 011-31-4360-15745.

The Maharishi Sthapatya Veda *Program*

Sthapatya comes from the word sthapana, which means "to establish." Veda means "knowledge." The Maharishi Sthapatya Veda program provides the knowledge of establishment—how to establish the self in pure consciousness, the source of all life, and how to establish one's environment in accord with all the laws of nature so that one always enjoys nature's support.

Maharishi Sthapatya Veda design is the most ancient and supreme system of country, town, village, and home planning in accord with natural law—connecting individual life with cosmic life, individual intelligence with cosmic intelligence, and creating ideal living conditions on earth where everyone will feel, "I am living in heaven."

Maharishi Mahesh Yogi has commented, "Because the individual is cosmic, everything about individual life should be in full harmony with cosmic life. Maharishi Sthapatya Veda design gives dimensions, formulas, and orientations to the buildings that will provide cosmic harmony and support to the individual for his peace, prosperity, and good health—daily life in accord with natural law, daily life in the evolutionary direction."

In response to the urgent worldwide need for people to have ideal working and living environments, Maharishi Global Construction, L.L.C. was established to offer consulting services in Maharishi Sthapatya Veda design principles to architects, designers and builders. Maharishi Global Construction is currently designing 435 Maharishi Vedic Centers, one in each Congressional district throughout the United States, as models of architecture in accord with natural law. These buildings will house all of Maharishi's programs for the development of consciousness and the creation of perfect health, including the treatment and cure of chronic disease. The company is also designing 50 in-residence Maharishi Vedic Medical Centers, one in each state, for the treatment of chronic disease through the Maharishi Vedic Approach to Health.

For more information on Maharishi Sthapatya Veda design:

In the United States:

Maharishi Global Construction, L.L.C.   515-472-9605
500 North Third Street, Suite 110
Fairfield, IA 52556
E-mail: recption@MGC-Vastu.com
Web site: http://www.MGC-Vastu.com

In Canada:

Maharishi Global Construction   613-565-8525
E-mail: mgc-can@ottawa.com
Web site: http://www.mgc-Vastu.com

Notes

[1] Maharishi Mahesh Yogi, *Maharishi Forum of Natural Law and National Law for Doctors* (India: Age of Enlightenment Publications, 1995), p. 16.

[2] *Celebrating Perfection in Education* (India: Age of Enlightenment Publications, 1997), p. 83.

[3] S. Nidich, P. Morehead, R. Nidich, D. Sands, and H. Sharma, "The Effect of the Maharishi Student Rasayana Food Supplement on Non-Verbal Intelligence," *Personality and Individual Differences*, vol. 15, No. 5 (1993), pp. 599-602.

[4] K.N. Kileepan, S.T. Varghese, J.D. Page, and D.J. Stechschulte, "Enhanced Lymphoproliferative Response, Macrophage-Mediated Tumor Cell Killing and Nitric Oxide Production After Ingestion of an Ayurvedic Drug (MAK-5)," *Biochemical Archives*, vol. 9 (1993), pp. 365-374.

[5] *Charaka Samhita*, Sharirasthana 4:13.

[6] John W. Zamarra, M.D., Robert H. Schneider, M.D., Italo Besseghini, M.D., Donald K. Robinson, M.S., and John W. Salerno, Ph.D., "Usefulness of the Transcendental Meditation program in the Treatment of Patients with Coronary Artery Disease," *The American Journal of Cardiology*, vol. 77 (1996), pp. 867-870.

[7] Maharishi Mahesh Yogi, *Maharishi Forum of Natural Law and National Law for Doctors* (India: Age of Enlightenment Publications, 1995), p. 53.

8 *Charaka Samhita,* Sharirasthana 2:46-47.

9 Robert Keith Wallace, "The Physiological Effects of *Transcendental Meditation," Science,* vol. 167 (1970), p. 1750.

10 K. Reddy, T. Egenes, and L. Egenes, *All Love Flows to the Self: Eternal Stories from the Upanishads* (Schenectady: Samhita Enterprises, 1998).

11 *Sushruta Samhita,* Sutrasthana 15: 41.

12 *Charaka Samhita,* Sharirasthana 6:18.

13 *Sushruta Samhita,* Sharirasthana 3:16.

14 *Charaka Samhita,* Sharirasthana 3:1-2.

15 *Charaka Samhita,* Sharirasthana 8:17.

16 *Charaka Samhita,* Sharirasthana 4:15.

17 *Sushruta Samhita,* Sharirasthana 3:32.

18 All references for the first eight months of life are from *Charaka Samhita,* Sharirasthana 4:9-26.

19 *Charaka Samhita,* Sharirasthana 6:22.

20 *Charaka Samhita,* Sharirasthana 6:23.

21 *Sushruta Samhita,* Sharirasthana 3:18.

22 *Charaka Samhita,* Vimanasthana 1:23.

23 *Charaka Samhita,* Sutrasthana 30:9-10.

24 *Charaka Samhita,* Vimanasthana 1:25-II.

25 See H. Sharma and C. Clark, *Contemporary Ayur-Veda* (New York: Churchill Livingstone, 1998), pp. 66-67

26 B.S. Nath and M.K. Rama Murthy, "Cholesterol in Indian Ghee," *Lancet,* vol. 2 (1988), p. 39.

27 Daniel Q. Harvey, "Cradle to grave, birth weight may matter," *Albany* (NY) *Times Union* (February 2, 1997)

28 *Charaka Samhita,* Sharirasthana 8:22.

29 *Sushruta Samhita,* Sharirasthana 3:12.

30 *Sushruta Samhita,* Sharirasthana 10:3.

31 *Sushruta Samhita,* Sharirasthana 10:3.

32 G. Rottman, "Untersuchengen uber Einstellung zur Schwangerschaft und zur fotalen Entwiklung," *Geist und Psyche,* H.

Graber, ed. (Munich: Kindler Verlag, 1974).

[33] R.L. Cohen in M. Klaus and J. Kennell, *Maternal-Infant Bonding* (St. Louis, MO: C.V. Mosby, 1976), p. 46.

[34] M. Lukesch in T. Verny, with J. Kelly, *The Secret Life of the Unborn Child* (New York: Summit, 1981), p. 49.

[35] D. Stott, "Children in the Womb: The Effects of Stress," *New Society* (May 19, 1977), pp. 329-331.

[36] *Charaka Samhita*, Sharirasthana 8:16.

[37] D. Retallack, *The Sound of Music and Plants* (Marina del Ray, CA: Devors and Company, 1973), pp. 20-23.

[38] J. Alvin, *Music Therapy* (London: John Baker Publishers, 1966).

[39] M.A. Bruya and B. Severtsen, "Evaluating the effects of music on electroencephalogram patterns of normal subjects," *Journal of Neurosurgical Nursing*, vol. 16, no. 2 (1984), pp. 96-100.

[40] H.M. Sharma, E. Kauffman, and R. Stephens, Alternative Therapies in Clinical Practice, vol. 3, no. 4 (1996), pp. 25–32.

[41] T. Verny, with J. Kelly, *The Secret Life of the Unborn Child* (New York: Summit Books, 1981), pp. 22-23.

[42] *Charaka Samhita*, Sharirasthana 8:38.

[43] *Charaka Samhita*, Sharirasthana 8:40.

[44] C. Brown, ed., "The Many Facets of Touch," *Johnson and Johnson Pediatric Round Table*, no. 10 (New York: Elsevier, 1984).

[45] *Sushruta Samhita*, Sharirasthana 10:4.

[46] R.P. Lederman, E. Lederman, B.A. Work, and D.S. McCann, "The Relationship of Maternal Anxiety, Plasma Catecholamines, and Plasma Cortisol to Progress in Labor," *American Journal of Obstetrics and Gynecology* (1978), pp. 132, 495-500.

[47] Marshall H. Klaus, "Touching During and After Childbirth," in *Touch in Early Development*, by Tiffany M. Field (Mahwah, NJ: Lawrence Erlbaum Associates, 1995), p. 30.

[48] M.H. Klaus and J.H. Kennel, *Maternal-Infant Bonding: The Impact of Early Separation or Loss on Family Development* (St. Louis: C.V. Mosby, 1976).

49 *Charaka Samhita,* Sharirasthana 8:49.

50 J.S. Brooks and T. Scarano, "Transcendental Meditation in the Treatment of Post-Vietnam Adjustment," *Journal of Counseling and Development,* vol. 65 (1985), pp. 212–215.

51 M. Biefeld, "TM: A Stress-Reducing Self-Help Support System," (Cleveland Veterans Administration Medical Center), presented at the Annual Meeting of the American Psychological Association (Los Angeles, CA), August 24, 1981.

52 Maharishi Forum for Natural Law and National Law for Doctors (Canada: Age of Enlightenment Publications, 1996) p. 52.

53 J.F. Clinton, "Physical and Emotional Responses of Expectant Fathers Throughout Pregnancy and the Early Postpartum Period," *International Journal of Nursing Studies,* vol. 24, no. 1 (1987), pp. 59-88.

54 D.D. Affonso and G. Domino "Postpartum Depression: A Review," *Birth,* vol. 24, no. 1 (1984), pp. 231-235.

55 T.G. Arizmendi, D.D. Affonso, and G. Domino, "Research on Psychological Factors and Postpartum Depression: A Critique," *Birth,* vol. 24, no. 1 (1984), pp. 237-245.

56 D.D. Affonso, "Assessment of Maternal Postpartum Adaptation," *Public Health Nursing,* vol. 4, no. 1 (1987), pp. 9-20.

57 V.L. Larsen, "Stresses of the Childbearing Year," *American Journal of Public Health,* vol. 56 (1966), pp. 32-36.

58 T.G. Arizmendi, D.D. Affonso, and G. Domino, "Research on Psychological Factors and Postpartum Depression: A Critique," *Birth,* vol. 24, no. 1 (1984), pp. 237-245.

59 J. Errante, "Sleep Deprivation or Postpartum Blues," *Topics in Clinical Nursing,* 6 (4) (1985), pp. 9-18.

60 C. Fakouri and P. Jones, "Relaxation Rx: Slow Stroke Back Rub," *Journal of Gerontological Nursing,* vol. 13 (1987), pp. 32-35.

61 S. Dunbar, "Should Patients with Acute Myocardial Infarctions Receive Back Massage?" *Focus Critical Care* (June 1986), pp. 42-46.

62 *Sushruta Samhita,* Sutrasthana 19:20.

[63] *Sushruta Samhita,* Sutrasthana 19:26.

[64] Robin Lim, *After the Baby's Birth: A Woman's Way to Wellness* (Berkeley, CA: Celestial Arts, 1991), p. 63.

[65] H. Sharma, A. Hanna, E. Kauffman, and H. Newman, "Inhibition of Human Low-Density Lipoprotein Oxidation in Vitro by Maharishi Ayur-Veda Herbal Mixtures MAK-4, MAK-5, MA-631, and Maharishi Coffee Substitute," Pharmacology, Biochemistry and Behavior, vol. 43 (1992), pp. 1175-1182.

[66] H.M. Sharma, Y. Feng, and R.V. Panganamala, "Maharishi Amrit Kalash (MAK) Prevents Human Platelet Aggregation," *Clinica & Terapia Cardiovascolare,* vol. 3 (1989), pp. 227-230.

[67] *Sushruta Samhita,* Sharirasthana 10:46-47.

[68] Ashley Montagu, *Touching: The Human Significance of the Skin* (New York: Harper and Row, 1986), pp. 4-5.

[69] D.E. Smith and J.W. Salerno, "Selective Growth Inhibition of a Human Malignant Melanoma Cell Line by Sesame Oil in Vitro," Prostaglandins, Leukotrines and Essential Fatty Acids, vol. 46 (1992), pp. 145-150.

[70] J.W. Salerno and D.E. Smith, "The Use of Sesame Oil and Other Vegetable Oils in the Inhibition of Human Colon Cancer Growth in Vitro," *Anticancer Research,* vol. 11 (1992), pp. 209-216.

[71] Teresa Kirkpatrick Ramsey, *Baby's First Massage* (Elma, New York: The International Association of Infant Massage, 1992), p. 15.

[72] Tiffany M. Field, Ph.D., et al., "Tactile/Kinesthetic Stimulation Effects on Preterm Neonates," *Pediatrics,* vol. 77, no. 5 (May 1986), p. 654-658.

[73] R. Rice, "Neurophysiological Development in Premature Infants Following Stimulation," *Developmental Psychology,* vol. 13 (1977).

[74] H. Epstein, "Phrenoblysis: Special Brain and Mind Growth Periods." *Developmental Psychology* (New York: Wiley, 1974).

[75] *Sushruta Samhita*, Sharirasthana 10:30.

[76] See Ashley Montagu, *Touching: The Human Significance of the Skin* (New York: Harper and Row, 1986), p. 75.

[77] Carl Jones, *After the Baby is Born: A Complete Postpartum Guide for New Parents*, (New York: Dodd, Mead & Company, 1986), p. 39.

[78] C. Hoefer and M.C. Hardy, "Later Development of Breast Fed and Artificially Fed Infants," *Journal of the American Medical Association*, vol. 96 (1929), pp. 615-619.

[79] F.M. Pottenger, Jr., "The Responsibility of the Pediatrician in the Orthodontic Problem," *California Medicine*, vol. 65 (1946), pp. 169-170.

[80] F.E. Broad, "Further Studies on the Effects of Infant Feeding on Speech Quality," *New Zealand Medical Journal*, vol. 82 (1975), pp. 373-376.

[81] K.R. Eppley, A.I. Abrams, and J. Shear, "Differential effects of relaxation techniques on trait anxiety: A meta-analysis," *Journal of Clinical Psychology*, vol. 45 (1989), pp. 957-974.

[82] Maharishi Mahesh Yogi, *Science of Being and Art of Living* (New York: Meridian, 1995), pp. 284-285.

[83] "Neonatal Separation: The Maternal Side of Interactional Deprivation," *Pediatrics*, vol. 54, no. 0 (1970), p. 197.

[84] John Bowlby, "Disruption of Affectional Bonds and Its Effects on Behavior," *Mental Health Supplement, Bimonthly Journal of the Department of National Health and Welfare*, Ottawa, Canada (January-February 1969).

[85] M.H. Klaus and J. Kennell, "Maternal Attachment: Importance of the First Post-Partum Days," *The New England Journal of Medicine*, vol. 286 (March 2, 1972), pp. 460-463.

[86] T.B. Brazelton and B.G. Cramer, *The Earliest Relationship* (Reading, MA: Addison-Wesley, 1990).

[87] M.H. Klaus and J.H. Kennel, *Parent-Infant Bonding* (St. Louis: Mosby, 1982).

[88] F. Stirnimann in F. Kruse, "Nos Souvenirs du Corps Maternel,"

Psychologie Heute (June 25, 1978) p. 56.

[89] Gail Peterson et al., "The Role of Some Birth-Related Variables in Father Attachment," *American Journal of Orthopsychiatry*, vol. 49, no. 2 (April 1979), pp. 330-338.

[90] Ibid., pp. 330-338.

[91] M. Greenberg and N. Morris, "Engrossment: The Newborn's Impact on the Father," *American Journal of Orthopsychiatry*, vol. 44 (1974), pp. 520-531.

[92] Montagu, op. cit., pp. 71-73.

[93] Montagu, op. cit., pp. 292-392.

[94] N.W. Johnson, "Breastfeeding in the First Hour of Life," *American Journal of Maternal-Child Nursing*, no. 1 (1976), pp. 12-16.

[95] Verny, with Kelly, op. cit., pp. 147-164.

[96] Montagu, op.cit., pp. 96-100.

[97] Montagu, op.cit., pp. 96-100.

[98] D. Goleman, "Patterns of Love Charted in Studies," *The New York Times* (Sept 10, 1985).

[99] M. Roberts, "Baby Love" [Effects of infant experience on later adult love life; a study by Shaver and Hazan], *Psychology Today* (March 1987)

[100] *Charaka Samhita*, Sharirasthana 8:64-66.

[101] C.A. Dixon, "Consciousness and Cognitive Development: A Six-Month Longitudinal Study of Four-Year-Olds Practicing the Children's Transcendental Meditation Technique," Doctoral Dissertation, Department of Psychology, Maharishi International University (1989).

Index

About the Authors

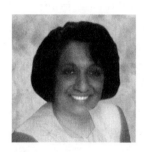

Kumuda Reddy, M.D.

Kumuda Reddy has practiced medicine for more than twenty years. She completed her residency and fellowship in anesthesiology at Mt. Sinai Hospital, New York.

Dr. Reddy is a former faculty member and anesthesiologist at Albany Medical College. She is currently an adjunct faculty member there, and directs the Maharishi Vedic Medical Center of Upstate New York. In addition to writing and lecturing extensively on Maharishi Vedic Medicine, Dr. Reddy writes books based on the traditional stories of India.

Dr. Reddy lives in Niskayuna, New York, with her husband Janardhan, a practicing urologist, and her three children, Sundeep, Suma, and Hima.

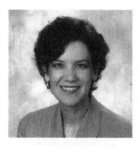

Linda Egenes, M.A.

Linda Egenes has written extensively about Maharishi Vedic Medicine for national magazines and newsletters. She also writes books for children. She teaches literary journalism at Maharishi University of Management in Fairfield, Iowa, where she lives with her husband Tom.

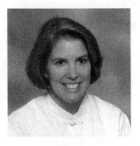

Margaret Mullins, MSN, CFNP

Margaret Mullins has her certification as a pediatric and family nurse practitioner, and has worked primarily in the areas of obstetric and pediatric nursing. She began working clinically with the Maharishi Vedic Approach to Health in 1985, and helped develop the Maharishi Ayur-Veda Mother and Baby program. She currently has her own practice as a nurse practitioner combining the Maharishi Vedic Approach to Health and allopathic medicine. The parents of 23-year-old twin daughters, she and her husband live in Boone, North Carolina.